'Bravo! The importance of movement skills has been ignored for too long. Dr Crawford's fundamental movement skills are a wake-up call to clinicians, psychologists and therapists caring for children and adults with ASD. Recognizing that FMS need to be learned, practiced and reinforced puts the responsibility on all of us to ensure children and adults with ASD have access to movement training. This book is a roadmap to better health, socialization and enjoyment of an active life.'

— *Judith H. Miles, MD, PhD, Thompson Center for Autism & Neurodevelopmental Disorders, University of Missouri Health Care*

'Accessible and individualized to meet every learner's needs, Susan Crawford ensures this book will benefit parents and professionals alike. A must read for anyone wanting to understand how to develop physical skills and a go-to book for people at all stages of their autism journey.'

— *Sharon McCarthy, parent, consultant and host of Autism Journeys Radio Show*

'For many years, Susan Crawford has inspired and continues to inspire many individuals in the world of ASD. This book provides credible teaching methodologies and tools that will practically guide and support those who value the importance of developing FMS in children and adults with ASD. What she has created in this book as well as her online website is a testament to her hard work and dedication. This will be my go-to-guide for many years to come when teaching FMS. I admire and take my hat off to Susan for creating this invaluable piece of work!'

— *Fiona O'Sullivan Downey, Cork Institute of Technology & University College Cork*

'Dr Crawford expertly presents the reader with the knowledge and skills required to successfully enhance the fundamental motor skills of children with autism. This book is comprehensive; drawing relevant theory from the fields of motor development, motor learning, health promotion and autism research. It will motivate, educate and empower the reader to get children with autism skillfully moving. It's a must-have for the practitioner's bookshelf!'

— Seán Healy, PhD, Assistant Professor of Behavioral Health and Nutrition, University of Delaware

'This book is an authentic, innovative and inspiring resource that has the potential to enhance the lives of individuals with ASD. Susan's passion and experience for this topic is evident throughout. Clear practical guidelines are provided on the assessment and promotion of FMS for ASD that are invaluable for parents, clinicians, teachers and coaches.'

— Dr Tom Comyns, Lecturer in Human Movement Science, University of Limerick

Fundamental Movement Skill Acquisition for Children and Adults with Autism

of related interest

Helping Children to Improve Their Gross Motor Skills
The Stepping Stones Curriculum
Rachel White
ISBN 978 1 78592 279 4
eISBN 978 1 78450 587 5

**The Parent's Guide to Occupational Therapy
for Autism and Other Special Needs**
Practical Strategies for Motor Skills, Sensory
Integration, Toilet Training, and More
Cara Koscinski
ISBN 978 1 78592 705 8
eISBN 978 1 78450 258 4

Autism Movement Therapy® Method
Waking Up the Brain!
Joanne Lara with Keri Bowers
Foreword by Stephen M. Shore
ISBN 978 1 84905 728 8
eISBN 978 1 78450 173 0

The Autism Fitness Handbook
An Exercise Program to Boost Body Image, Motor Skills, Posture and
Confidence in Children and Teens with Autism Spectrum Disorder
David S. Geslak
ISBN 978 1 84905 998 5
eISBN 978 0 85700 963 0

**Understanding Motor Skills in Children with Dyspraxia,
ADHD, Autism, and Other Learning Disabilities**
A Guide to Improving Coordination
Lisa A. Kurtz
ISBN 978 1 84310 865 8
eISBN 978 1 84642 672 8

Fundamental Movement Skill Acquisition for Children and Adults with Autism

A Practical Guide to Teaching and Assessing Individuals on the Spectrum

Dr SUSAN CRAWFORD PhD

Foreword by David Sugden

Jessica Kingsley *Publishers*
London and Philadelphia

First published in 2018
by Jessica Kingsley Publishers
73 Collier Street
London N1 9BE, UK
and
400 Market Street, Suite 400
Philadelphia, PA 19106, USA

www.jkp.com

Library of Congress Cataloging in Publication Data
Names: Crawford, Susan (Susan Margaret), author.
Title: Fundamental movement skill acquisition for children and adults with
    autism : a practical guide to teaching and assessing individuals on the
    spectrum / Susan Crawford.
Description: London ; Philadelphia : Jessica Kingsley Publishers, 2018. |
    Includes bibliographical references.
Identifiers: LCCN 2018002487 | ISBN 9781785923722
Subjects: LCSH: Movement education. | Movement disorders. | Autistic
    children--Education. | Autism spectrum disorders--Treatment.
Classification: LCC RC489.D3 C73 2018 | DDC 616.85/882--dc23 LC
record available at https://catalog.loc.gov/vwebv/search?
searchCode=LCCN&searchArg=2018002487&searchType=1&permalink=y

British Library Cataloguing in Publication Data
A CIP catalogue record for this book is available from the British Library

ISBN 978 1 78592 372 2
eISBN 978 1 78450 716 9

Printed and bound in the United States

Dedicated to

Tomás,

with all my love.

In memory of Dr P.J. Smyth (RIP):

For many years of great friendship, teaching,
inspiration, mentorship and support.

Contents

Foreword

In writing this foreword I have looked at three aspects the book either directly or tacitly covers. The first one concerns the importance of movement in everyday life for all; the second focuses on the condition known as autism spectrum disorder (ASD) and the third looks at the experience and skill of the author.

First, movement, occasionally neglected by psychologists and others in favour of cognitions or language, is the one and only ability we have that interacts with other humans, animals and the environment. We learn to move and we move in order to learn. One has only to think about and list what one does from getting up in the morning to going to bed at night and think of any activity (maybe thinking!) that does not involve movement. It is fundamental to our lives, and early locomotive skills act as a catalyst for other abilities such as perception, memory and cognitions. From these, ideas such as 'embodied cognition' have taken a similar stance. Movement always operates in contexts and, as such, the unit of analysis is never just the individual: it is the individual taught in a particular way in a particular environment, with the triad and dynamic transactions of these variables all being important. They contribute to the individual being able to engage and participate and learn. This book embodies the philosophy of movement enhancing daily life activities in appropriate contexts; it emphasises the importance of movement and shows how lives are improved through the capability of movement. Of note is the theme that theoretical and practical aspects of movement programmes are two sides of the same coin and join to provide solid evidence for the work.

Second, we now know so much more about individuals with ASD. We know that they perceive the world in a different manner to the rest of us, and have a different frame of reference. They are not necessarily negative, and indeed many show extraordinary abilities in certain fields, but they do differ, and it is these differences we need to cater for in order to release their potential. They have some challenges but also huge positives, which if corralled by helpful others, can enhance their lives significantly. Movement is one of these, and one has only to watch, as I have done, movement programmes for individuals with ASD and the positives that arise from them to recognise the benefits. In addition to the joy and success these individuals gain from fundamental movement skills such as running and jumping and other locomotor activities leading to social games, they also gain in confidence and competence, and, through movement, learn such skills as cooperation and even competition if organised appropriately. We have much evidence to show that movement enhances their daily lives, and this book shows how this can be done.

Finally, the author: Susan Crawford. I first came across Susan when I was external examiner for her undergraduate degree. I had to interview her as she was on course for a first class honours degree, a target she easily accomplished. Subsequently, I watched her complete her very fine PhD. One can examine how she has operated in three different yet interrelated roles: as an academic and clinician, a leader and a mother. As an academic and clinician she brings rigour to all of her work. She cites evidence that is based on theoretical substrates, empirical data and, last but not least, professional clinical practice, of which hers is a stand-out example. As a leader, she has a rare ability to corral speakers, experts, administrators, families and others, and give a sense of ownership and empowerment to those who have been neglected over the years. Through this she has made important contributions to the overall wellbeing of children with ASD. Third, over a 20-year period I have watched her as a mother support, care for and raise her beloved Tomás. She has done this with untiring devotion, with protection, with support, but also with pragmatics. She shows her love and devotion by her kindness and care, but also in teaching Tomás the pragmatic skills necessary for successful everyday functioning. In the field of movement and ASD I know of no other person who can bring this kind of experience, skill and love to the subject.

Emeritus Professor David Sugden
University of Leeds

Acknowledgements

My heartfelt thanks to the many children and adults with autism spectrum disorder (ASD), to their parents and to their practitioners, who have inspired me along this particular journey. Equally, I would like to acknowledge those influential researchers, teachers, occupational therapists, physiotherapists, sports performers and lecturers who have contributed to our ever-growing knowledge of the importance of developing quality movement skills for both individuals with ASD and the general population. In particular, I would like to pay tribute to two wonderful motor psychologists, Dr P.J. Smyth (RIP) and Professor David Sugden, who have changed the trajectory of fundamental movement skill education and training both here in Ireland and internationally.

I wish to acknowledge the many undergraduate students and graduates of our Sports Studies and Physical Education Degree programme in University College Cork, Ireland, who have contributed to the development and delivery of both quality fundamental movement skills programmes and physical activity programmes for children and adults of varying abilities across communities.

Thanks to the members of Health Action Zone, Health Service Executive (HSE), Cork, Ireland, for collaborating and supporting the development of fundamental movement skills, physical activity and health-related resources and programmes for children and adults in our communities. I especially wish to acknowledge Bernard Twomey, Stephen Murphy and Martin Aherne of Health Action Zone, HSE, Cork, Ireland, who have worked with me tirelessly on all our initiatives and helped ensure these programmes meaningfully came to fruition.

Thank you to the Irish Research Council of Science, Engineering and Technology (IRCSET), the Fulbright Commission and University College Cork's major Grant Application Fund for supporting my research in the field of ASD. I would also like to acknowledge Dr Maire Leane at University College Cork for her ongoing mentoring, support and belief in this work.

Finally, I wish to acknowledge my wonderful son Tomás, who has inspired me to walk where I might have feared to go.

Dr Susan Crawford, PhD
University College Cork, Ireland

Introduction

Addressing fundamental movement skills for children and adults on the autistic spectrum is an essential component to promoting quality of life issues for this particular population. Fundamental movement skills are those skills of movement that we often take for granted in everyday life. These include walking, running, jumping, hopping, balance, throwing and catching, to mention but a few. For the general population these movement skills do not develop to maturity without appropriate practice. Lack of maturity in fundamental movement skills has been associated with reduced participation in sport-specific skills, physical inactivity and the development of health-related complications associated with sedentary lifestyles. Equally, the benefits of participation in physical activity for emotional and social development across the lifespan are well documented. Participants have the opportunity to engage with others, develop social networks and to enjoy the feelings of wellbeing associated with quality movement.

Delay and impairment in fundamental movement skill development for children and adults on the autistic spectrum have been established. However, programmes to address fundamental movement skill delay for this population have proven successful when implemented with appropriate support and training. Parents, educationalists, clinical therapists and others often feel overwhelmed when trying to address these concepts. This book provides a step-by-step approach to addressing fundamental movement skill development for children and adults with autism spectrum disorder (ASD). The book also includes an in-depth exploration of programme planning, implementation and evaluation using empirically validated teaching and learning methodologies. The book is supported by an online resource: www.getautismactive.com. The online resource provides complementary video guidelines, voiceover instruction and a checklist for each movement skill. Suggestions for incidental teaching and learning are also included. This approach to embracing the 'learning to move, moving to learn' philosophy for children and adults with ASD opens doors for overall growth and development in health and wellbeing across the lifespan, and is accessible to all.

Outline of the book

Chapter 1 Introduction to Autism Spectrum Disorder: This chapter sets the scene, exploring the diagnosis of ASD, considers Diagnostic and Statistical Manual of Mental Disorders, Fifth Edition (DSM-5; American Psychiatric Association, 2013) criteria and introduces theories associated with the condition. Issues to consider in relation to ASD are presented. The prevalence of ASD and associated conditions are included. The final section outlines teaching and learning methodologies particularly used in relation to fundamental movement skill development for individuals on the spectrum.

Chapter 2 Introduction to Fundamental Movement Skills: This chapter explores the principles and practice of fundamental movement skills (FMS) development. The chapter opens with a definition of motor development, and goes on to explain the phases and stages of FMS development from *in utero* to adulthood. The importance of developing FMS is explained from a research perspective. The factors that contribute to FMS development are introduced, as is the facilitation of FMS from initial to mature stages of development. The importance of observation and programme planning is explored. Sections on the use of demonstration and feedback are included. An explanation of closed and open motor skills is provided. The chapter leads on to an exploration of the domains of learning. Concepts of assessment are introduced and the chapter closes with a selection of mature FMS including voiceover prompts, identifying features and links to the skill being visually demonstrated on the www.getautismactive.com website.

Chapter 3 Exploring ASD and Fundamental Movement Skill Research: Chapter 3 considers some research studies in relation to motor impairment and fundamental movement skill interventions for individuals with ASD. A section on research reporting physical activity levels of individuals with ASD is included.

Chapter 4 Tools for Assessment of Fundamental Movement Skills of individuals with ASD: This chapter considers some of the assessment tools used in relation to assessing fundamental movement skills for individuals with ASD. These include the Movement Assessment Battery for Children (Henderson and Sugden, 1992; Henderson, Sugden and Barnett 2007a, 2007b); the Peabody Developmental Motor Scales – Second Edition (PDMS-2) (Folio and Fewell, 1983, 2000); the Test of Gross Motor Development 2 (Ulrich, 1985, 2000); the Bruininks–Osteretsky Test of Motor Proficiency (BOTMP-BOT2) (Bruininks, 1978); and the Manchester Motor Skills Assessment (MMSA) (Bond et al., 2007). The Reflective Framework for Teaching and Learning in Physical Education (Tsangaridou and O'Sullivan, 1994) has been included as a useful qualitative tool.

Chapter 5 Promoting and Maintaining Participation in Fundamental Movement Skill Programmes for Individuals with ASD: This chapter provides guidelines on programme assessment, planning, design and implementation for this population. The chapter explores understanding of the individual, the environment and the task being planned.

Intervention and programme planning for individuals with ASD consider individual instruction, low student to teacher ratio, task variation, and stimulus generalisation of learning, self-determination, structured learning environment and physical structure. The ASD/FMS support kit identifies some useful backup tools for programme planning and delivery. The final section on how to maximise skill acquisition is supported in each aspect with case scenarios from parents or practitioners in the field. This includes allowing time for familiarity, promoting eye contact, use of clear language, being aware of sensory preferences and overselectivity, balancing social skills training and physical activity, objectives, the use of Applied Behaviour Analysis, the use of recording format, the use of prompts, the use of reinforcements, the use of incidental teaching, the use of pivotal response training, the use of Treatment and Education of Autistic and related Communication Handicapped Children (TEACCH) components, the use of Mobile Digital Technology (MDT)/video analysis, and the use of proprioceptive stretches pre- and post-FMS programme.

Chapter 6 www.getautismactive.com: Bringing it All Together: Chapter 6 explores getautismactive, the online programme for addressing fundamental movement skill development for individuals on the spectrum (www.getautismactive.com).

Conclusions and Future Directions Identified: The book closes with some thoughts on how the agenda of ASD and FMS might be driven from research, policy and practice perspectives.

Introduction to Autism Spectrum Disorder

Historically, autism spectrum disorder (ASD) was identified as far back as the 1800s. The condition became more definitively established after the publication of research from the 1940s, including the work of Kanner (1943), Asperger (1944) and others. Since then, diagnostic criteria, issues, theories and causes of ASD have continued to evolve. Chapter 1 sets the scene and examines current diagnostic criteria, prevailing issues, theories, prevalence, causes and conditions associated with ASD. This chapter also considers interventions for children and adults with ASD that are especially relevant to developing quality movement experiences.

Diagnosis of ASD

This section includes:

- Autism being a spectrum disorder

- The triad of impairments

- The importance of comprehensive diagnosis

- Diagnostic and Statistical Manual of Mental Disorders Fifth Edition (DSM-5) and the International Classification of Diseases Tenth Revision (ICD-10) (World Health Organization, 1992)

- Differential diagnosis between DSM-IV and DSM-5

- Concerns about DSM-5

In 1996, Lorna Wing, the renowned UK-based psychiatrist, ASD researcher and, indeed, mother of a child with a diagnosis of autism, presented the notion of ASD being a spectrum disorder. She identified the condition as having a common triad of impairments, notably difficulties in social understanding, difficulties in social communication, and a lack of flexibility of thoughts and behaviours. Further variations of the condition included autistic disorder, Asperger's disorder, high functioning ASD and pervasive developmental disorder – not otherwise specified (PDD-NOS). So what differentiated these conditions? Autistic disorder involved a child being diagnosed with both ASD and learning disability. Asperger's disorder and high functioning ASD included children with a diagnosis of ASD but with an above average IQ who did not display language delay. A diagnosis of PDD-NOS was typically applied to children with some features of ASD but not all of the entire diagnostic criteria. In her work, Wing indicated that a diagnosis of ASD was usually made by recognising patterns of behaviour present from early in life. She also stressed the importance of compiling a detailed personal history with parents, which should include the history of development from infancy and a clear description of current behaviours. Wing advocated that an experienced psychologist should carry out the psychological assessment as soon as possible after issues arising, using a range of appropriate tests accompanied by questions designed specifically to diagnose ASD.

Since then, our understanding of ASD has grown. Currently, the two main systems for diagnosis are the Diagnostic and Statistical Manual of Mental Disorders (DSM), edited by the American Psychiatric Association, and the International Classification of Diseases (ICD-10), published by the World Health Organization. The DSM-IV was replaced by the DSM-5 in 2013. The DSM-5 presented a new classification of ASD and a revision of the criteria for diagnosis (2013), which attracted some public disquiet. The ICD-10 update was scheduled for release in late 2017/early 2018, but at the time of publication is still under consideration. An exploration of the DSM-5 revision is worthwhile as it helps us to better grasp what is now understood by the term autism spectrum disorder or ASD.

The revised diagnostic criteria for ASD in the DSM-5 (American Psychiatric Association, 2013) consider that deficits exist in both social communication and social interaction that are persistent in different contexts. The criteria also include the presence of repetitive behaviour, activity and interest patterns. These symptoms must be present during typical child development periods and will often present in a more definitive manner when social demands are great and when learned coping skills cannot address these demands. The DSM-5 identifies that these symptoms can cause serious impairment in different aspects of activities of everyday living and are not identifiable as an intellectual disability.

So how does this differ from the DSM-IV? The DSM-IV (APA, 1994) defined ASD and related disorders as 'pervasive developmental disorders' (PDDs). This definition has been replaced with the term 'autism spectrum disorders' (ASDs), which are included in the 'neurodevelopmental disorders' category. In the DSM-IV classification, the category of pervasive developmental disorders included the five different subtypes of ASD as outlined previously: autistic disorder, Asperger's disorder, childhood disintegrative disorder, pervasive developmental disorder – not otherwise specified (PDD-NOS) and Rett syndrome. The DSM-5 has replaced four of these subtypes with one main diagnosis, 'autism spectrum disorder' (ASD). Rett syndrome is no longer included. The DSM-5 specifies three levels of symptom severity and the intensity of support needed for ASD. The diagnostic definition of ASD in the DSM-IV was characterised by three core symptoms that made up the triad of impairments and included impaired social reciprocity, impaired language/communication, and restricted and repetitive pattern of interests/activities. In the DSM-5, there are now just two symptom categories: 'social communication deficits' (combining social and communication problems) and 'restricted/repetitive behaviours'. 'Language impairment/ delay' is no longer included in this symptom category, and a new clinical feature 'unusual sensitivity to sensory stimuli' has been incorporated into repetitive behaviours. A further change is that the diagnostic criterion of onset of ASD before 36 months of age is replaced with 'Symptoms must be present in early childhood, but may not become fully manifest until social demands exceed limited capacities'. The DSM-5 introduces a new diagnostic label within the category of 'language impairments' of 'social communication disorder'. The diagnostic features of this category partially overlap with that of ASD, as children diagnosed with social communication disorder are required to have an 'impairment of pragmatics' as well as impairment in the 'social uses of verbal and nonverbal communication'. However, the additional presence of fixated interests and repetitive behaviours excludes the possibility of a diagnosis of social communication disorder. Therefore, the occurrence of repetitive behaviours is essential for the differential diagnosis of ASD.

In their review, Vivanti *et al.* (2013) considered some of the criticisms of the DSM-5. These authors indicated that the most common criticism of the DSM-5 definition of ASD was that the new criteria were too narrow and could lead to some individuals being excluded from a diagnosis of ASD and subsequent access to services. Concerns about the new diagnosis of social communication disorder were also raised as access to relevant treatment for this condition might be difficult.

Again concerns about Asperger's disorder no longer being a separate condition were considered, as possibly affecting the identity of those previously diagnosed with the condition. However, the counter-argument to that was that often such a diagnosis led to affected people not being given access to support on the basis that they were high functioning. The term autism spectrum disorder (ASD) will be adopted hereafter throughout this textbook for consistency.

KEY POINTS

* Autism is now replaced with ASD, with all subtypes including Asperger's disorder replaced.

* ASD has two categories of impairment instead of three so a triad of impairments is replaced by a dyad of impairments, namely 'social communication deficits' (combining social and communication problems) and 'restricted/repetitive behaviours'.

* 'Language impairment/delay' is no longer included and a new clinical feature, 'unusual sensitivity to sensory stimuli', has been introduced.

* The diagnostic criterion of onset of ASD spectrum disorders before 36 months of age is replaced and allows for the condition not becoming obvious until social demands exceed the ability of the child to cope.

Exploring issues in the world of ASD

This section includes:

* Difficulties in social development

* Difficulties in language

* Difficulties in cognition

* Difficulties in motor mannerisms

- Sensory information processing

- Anxiety

- Behaviour issues

There are no behaviours per se that by their presence or absence indicate autism; it is the overall pattern and underlying difficulties that define autism.

(Jordan, Jones and Murray, 1998, p.14)

For the child and adult with ASD, difficulties may occur in areas of social development and are described as atypical (Wing, 2002). Issues in this area can include a lack of engagement and interest in people, delayed or inconsistent eye contact, and limited facial expressions and body language. These skills may or may not develop over time. Impairment may occur in both verbal and non-verbal communication and the acquisition of gestured communication skills (Seal and Bonvillian, 1997). Expressive and receptive language abilities are often delayed or disordered: verbally able individuals with ASD can be literal, pedantic and repetitive. Pragmatic skills can also be affected.

ASD can present with rigidity in both cognition and behaviour. Delayed development of play skills may present early on in childhood where stereotypical handling or arranging of objects, for example, lining up toys, can predominate over imaginative play. Autistic mannerisms including stereotypical behaviours can be a feature of the condition (Constantino and Gruber, 2005). Changes in routines and surroundings can cause a high degree of distress to individuals with ASD (Jordan, Jones and Murray, 1998). Preoccupations can develop with particular objects and routines.

Repetitive motor mannerisms and adherence to behaviour routines are commonplace (Wing, 2002). These movements can be associated with excitement, agitation or anger (Wing, 2002; Frith, 2003). Abnormalities of gait and posture may also occur.

Children with ASD often walk with shoulders and head bent forward, and often climb steps without alternating feet. Difficulties can occur with fine and gross motor movements (Ghaziuddin and Butler, 1998; Reid and Collier, 2002). This is further reflected in participation in physical activities and games. Individuals on the spectrum often prefer individual rather than team sports, as planning and organising movement can prove difficult. Children with ASD often have difficulty imitating movements, which further impairs social behaviour.

Reid and Collier (2002) have indicated that an examination of movement behaviour of individuals with ASD in empirical literature has supported delayed, average or precocious movement skills in ASD compared to their typically developed peers. Research confirming difficulties in motor development has provided a more definitive conclusion. Earlier studies of Berkeley *et al.* (2001) further confirmed these findings when comparing children with ASD to those who were typically developed. This topic will be examined in detail in Chapter 3.

Difficulties in processing sensory information have also been highlighted. Hyper- and hyposensitivity to sounds, visual information, patterns or movement, touch, textures, changes in temperature, odour and taste can occur. Manifestations of hyposensitivity can include staring intensely at lights, patterns and objects, listening to certain sounds and vibrations close to the ear, being unreactive to pain and injury, liking very strong smells and enjoyment of strong tastes (Grandin, 1996). Moving between hypo- and hypersensitivity has also been reported. Behaviours related to sensory perceptual difficulties include being able to process information from just one sensory channel at a time, having a fragmented perception of objects, people and situations, being easily distracted, and withdrawing as they go into sensory overload (Wing, 2002).

Anxiety can be an issue among individuals with ASD. This often arises in new or different situations, which they cannot understand. Wing (2002) indicated that individuals with ASD often do not understand real dangers, are calm when others are anxious and vice versa. Temple Grandin, a well-known author with ASD, wrote of fears of harmless items for no apparent reason.

The individual with ASD usually engages well in activities of interest to him or herself (Wing, 2002). However, in activities that are not motivating to the individual, the attention span can be short. Research has indicated that children with ASD can become easily distracted and find it hard to concentrate and complete the task at hand.

Some individuals with ASD develop special skills and aptitudes at different tasks (Frith, 2003; Howlin, 1997). Visuo-spatial skills not requiring language are often better developed than those skills that require speech (Wing, 2002). Many skills are often associated with repetitive action, for example, playing music.

Much has been written about the behaviour of children and adults with ASD (Crawford, MacDonncha and Smyth, 2007, 2013; Frith, 2003; Jordan *et al.*, 1998; Reid and O'Connor, 2003; Wing, 2002). Functions of inappropriate behaviours were identified as including the need for help or attention, escaping from stressful situations or activities, obtaining desired objects, protesting against unwanted events and obtaining stimulation (Frith, 2003; Reid and Collier, 2002; Wing, 2002). Behaviours can range from tantrums in public to touching or kissing a stranger (Wing, 2002).

Children and adults with ASD may seek out deep pressure manifested by deep hugs, leaning against walls or doors and excessively heavy footsteps when moving. This is often associated with the need for high levels of proprioceptive feedback (Crawford *et al.*, 2013).

KEY POINTS

* Difficulties in social development owing to lack of eye contact, social skills and play skills.

* Difficulties in language: may have verbal or non-verbal skills.

* Difficulties in cognition: may have difficulties of understanding.

* Difficulties in stereotypical mannerisms: may have repetitive behaviours.

* Difficulties in motor skills: may have problems with movement and balance.

* Sensory information processing issues: may have difficulty with different sensory issues.

* Anxiety: may get anxious with changes, especially in routines.

* Behaviour issues: may have behaviour issues such as agitation or tantrums.

Theories associated with ASD

This section includes:

* Mind blindness hypothesis

* Difficulties of weak central coherence

* Absence of a high level of control or action

Theories associated with ASD include the mind blindness hypothesis, difficulties of weak central coherence and absence of a high level of control or action. The mind blindness theory indicates a lack of understanding of the psychological health and wellbeing of other people. For individuals with high levels of functioning, this is overcome to some degree by compensatory learning, where individuals are then capable of manipulating and attributing mental states to others. The theory of weak central coherence indicates that individuals with ASD have a preference for a style of information processing that is focused on detail. An absence of higher-level control of action and attention indicates a difficulty in the self-organisation of any behaviour that is not routine, which is often attributed to stereotypical behaviours and narrow interests.

KEY POINTS

* Mind blindness: lack of understanding of others.

* Can focus on aspects of information.

* Preference for routine due to self-organisation difficulties.

Prevalence of ASD

This section includes:

* Incidence of ASD

* Associated learning disability

Over the past 30 years, the number of reported cases of ASD has increased in all countries where prevalence studies have been conducted. This increase is thought to be the result of increased awareness of ASD among health care professionals, parents and the broader population, changes to the diagnostic criteria for ASD, children being diagnosed at a younger age, and demographic and geographical variables. Given that prevalence studies vary in their scientific method, most are based on a limited sample of a country's population, rather than on national statistics. However, in a systematic review by Elsabbagh *et al.* (2012), a prevalence rate of 0.62 in 100 was reported globally. A prevalence study by Baird *et al.* in 2006 indicated that approximately one third of children with ASD also have a diagnosed learning disability. The US Centers for Disease Control and Prevention (2009) attribute this to the changed diagnostic criteria showing a scattered cognitive profile, and report the prevalence rate to be 1 in 65.

KEY POINTS

* Increased incidence.

* Prevalence rate of 0.62 in 100 globally.

* One third of children also have a learning disability.

* Prevalence rate in US of 1 in 65.

Causes of ASD

This section includes:

* Causes of ASD

* Twin studies

Despite many differing theories, the cause of ASD still remains unclear. In Kanner's earliest writing (1943) he considered ASD to be 'a constitutionally determined developmental disorder, primarily affecting social and emotional understanding'. He later wrote that the condition might be a response to dysfunctional patterns of family interaction. Subsequently, for decades parents were viewed as the cause of their children's disability. However, empirical investigations over time have provided no support for such views.

Folstein and Rutter (1977) published the first ASD twin study, indicating some evidence of a genetic base for ASD in identical twins. Frith (2003) indicated that the risk of a sibling being affected by a form of ASD has been estimated at 3–6 per cent, compared to a normal population risk of 0.6 per cent, making the risk of a second child being affected 5–10 times higher. By 2001, several researchers had completed genetic screens that identified several genomic regions containing genes that could be associated with ASD (National Alliance for Autism Research, 2005). However, genetic research is still ongoing. Today, there is growing evidence of genetic, neurobiological and environmental links to the condition.

KEY POINTS

* ASD has genetic, neurobiological and environmental links.

* There is a higher incidence in identical twins.

Conditions associated with ASD

This section includes:

*   Conditions that may occur with ASD

ASD can occur together with any other disability, physical or psychological. Individuals with ASD can also have other developmental disorders, such as attention deficit hyperactive disorder, dyslexia and developmental coordination disorder. They are also at higher risk of epilepsy, anxiety, depression and autism-related catatonia, particularly as they get older.

KEY POINTS

* ASD can occur with other developmental disorders.

* Those with ASD are at a higher risk of epilepsy, anxiety, depression and catatonia.

Teaching and learning interventions for individuals with ASD

This section includes:

- Teaching and learning interventions

- TEACCH

- Applied Behaviour Analysis

- Picture Exchange Communication System

- Pivotal Response Therapy

- Mobile Digital Technology

As ASD has evolved to a condition with no known cause or cure, a number of interventions have been developed to address different behaviours and characteristics that emerge, and indeed re-emerge, for individuals with a definitive diagnosis. These interventions are often designed to suit the learning style of the individual with ASD. This section outlines some of these in detail, in particular those used to address issues of difficulties in movement impairment. These include Treatment and Education of Autistic and related Communication Handicapped Children (TEACCH), Applied Behaviour Analysis (ABA), the Picture Exchange Communication System (PECS), Pivotal Response Therapy (PRT) and Mobile Digital Technology (MDT). These interventions can be classified according to the particular approach they adopt. ABA, PECS and PRT are considered behaviourist in approach. TEACCH and the use of MDT follow a more eclectic model, incorporating cognitive, behavioural and ecological elements. Many other interventions exist, but there is often little research evidence for their effectiveness.

TEACCH

TEACCH was founded by Eric Schopler in 1966 (cited in Schopler and Mesibov, 1986). The basic components of TEACCH include behavioural, developmental and ecological theoretical frameworks. The major approach of TEACCH is that of using a structured learning environment in order to learn new skills. Behavioural difficulties are viewed as the result of an individual's inability to understand and to cope with his or her environment. Hence, visual skills and routines are used to create meaningful environments. TEACCH promotes the involvement of the parents as co-therapists so that interventions can be implemented at home. In general, the programme provides a lifelong continuum of services including assessment and diagnosis, individualised treatment procedures, special education, social skills and vocational training, consultation, community collaboration and family support services (Erba, 2000).

Given the nature of the condition of ASD, clutter-free environments, structured visual schedules, task breakdown and generalisation of skills are all positive aspects of this approach. Generalised learning can occur and behaviour issues can be addressed simultaneously. Further, parents and professionals can access training in the TEACCH methodology locally, nationally and internationally (Jordan *et al.*, 1998).

ABA

The field of ABA is the scientific study of behaviour (Skinner, 1953). The work of Ivar Lovaas (1987, 1993) and Catherine Maurice (1993) helped established the efficacy of ABA as an ASD intervention from the late 1980s. In relation to ASD, the approach works in a systematic manner where each behaviour is measured in relation to the frequency or duration of its occurrence, what causes it to happen, what are appropriate reinforcers and generalisation of new skills. From a practical perspective, skills are broken down into component parts, a cue/antecedent is presented, a prompt may be introduced, reinforcers are given when the target response has occurred, opportunities to generalise responses are provided, and data from each performance are recorded and graphed. Active family participation is key to the successful delivery of an ABA programme, and home-based programmes have proven very successful (Dillenburger *et al.*, 2004).

Sample of a skill breakdown into component parts
Ball bouncing

- Feet are placed in narrow strike position, with opposite foot forward.

- Slight forward trunk lean.

- Ball is held waist high.

- Ball is pushed towards the ground, with follow-through of arm, wrist and fingers.

- There is controlled force of downward thrust.

- Repeated contact and pushing action is initiated from the fingertips.

- Visual monitoring is unnecessary.

- Controlled dribbling occurs.

Ball bouncing simplified

- Stand ready to bounce with the ball in one hand.

- Step forward with the opposite foot.

- Lean forward.

- Hold the ball at your waist.

- Bounce the ball.

- Push down hard with your hand.

- Repeat each time as the ball comes back.

- Try and get the 'feel' for the bounce.

- There is no need to watch or look at the ball.

- Repeat the ball bouncing with rhythm.

PECS

PECS was developed by Bondy and Frost in 1994, with the aim of enabling children with ASD and other communication deficits to acquire key communication skills in a social exchange. The PECS programme mainly combines prompting, reinforcement, error correction strategies and fading of prompts (Bondy and Frost, 2001; National Autistic Society, 2000). The programme starts with the child and two trainers initiating picture exchange, one responding to the child and the other providing as much physical prompting as necessary. Motivating stimuli such as toys, food and activities are used in order to build requesting. This further develops to labelling and using language (Quill, 2000).

The child moves from single-item pictures to construct a two-picture sentence, and therefore the social approach necessary for communication is further enhanced. The system moves from requesting to commenting as the child becomes more engaged in the process and the exchange.

PRT

PRT also embraces the principles of ABA. However, PRT focuses on pivotal behaviours (e.g. motivation) that when targeted, produce positive change in other (untargeted) areas of functioning and responding (Koegel and Koegel, 2006; Koegel, Koegel and Carter, 1999). It is the 'difficult to teach skills' that are targeted in PRT (Koegel and Koegel, 2006). PRT uses discrete trials including clear instructions, prompts and reinforcement. However, what is unique about PRT is that multiple behaviours are targeted at the same time and the reinforcements used are already found within the context of the task, making the interaction more natural and meaningful. Games and activities are considered part of natural interaction, along with turn taking, throwing and social communication. PRT is not about providing the child with a specific stimulus to respond to, but rather about creating multiple opportunities for them to initiate interaction, and essentially making them want to communicate and connect with others (Koegel et al., 1999). Four specific pivotal areas are targeted with PRT: (a) motivation to engage; (b) responding to multiple cues; (c) social initiation; and (d) self-regulation (Koegel and Koegel, 2006). PRT aims to motivate children with ASD to become increasingly responsive to everyday stimuli, and tries to make these everyday activities intrinsically motivating.

The primary teaching techniques advocated for in PRT to target motivation are: (a) the provision of choice; (b) providing direct and natural reinforcements; (c) rewarding attempts; and (d) interspersing acquisition and maintenance tasks (Koegel and Koegel, 2006). While all of these techniques are fundamental characteristics of quality teaching, it is the consistent use of them across all learning opportunities and the structuring of the environment to create these learning opportunities that make PRT effective. Some degree of choice can be integrated into almost any activity (Crawford et al., 2013). By providing choice in terms of activities, task goals or even the equipment they use, educators will learn what is meaningful to the children and adolescents with ASD, allowing them to be involved in and take ownership of their learning (Koegel et al., 1999). Furthermore, the provision of choice is likely to increase (intrinsic) interest in the activity (Koegel, Dyer and Bell, 1987) and provide motivation for continued participation.

MDT/video analysis

The use of video analysis and MDT is becoming more commonplace in relation to developing learning opportunities in the world of sport and physical education (Crawford, Lee and Fitzpatrick, 2015). It has also been found to be effective for individuals with ASD, particularly in programme planning for movement (Crawford *et al.*, 2013; Neely *et al.*, 2013). Video of environments, tasks, people, etc. can be created for individual programmes. These are then used to prepare the individual on the spectrum to participate in a programme, as a communication tool before, during and after each session, and as a record of progress. Video of skills can be used *in situ* as a teaching and learning tool as per the 'getautismactive' programme (www.getautismactive.com). This approach incorporates visual guidance, voiceover prompts and written instruction. It also includes opportunity for incidental teaching and learning. The programme is explored in detail later.

KEY POINTS

* Teaching and learning interventions are chosen to suit each learner.

* TEACCH: uses structure, visual aids and skill breakdown.

* ABA: uses skill breakdown, repetition and rewards.

* PECS: uses picture exchange and reward.

* PRT: uses choice, reinforcement, rewards, repetition.

* MDT: uses visual aids, video, iPads, mobile devices.

Summary

Chapter 1 introduced ASD and provided an exploration of the current DSM-V diagnostic criteria, with the two key criteria identified as social communication deficits, and restrictive and repetitive behaviours. This chapter also considered some of the issues – for example, social communication, repetitive behaviours and mannerisms, etc. – that may arise for individuals on the spectrum. Existing theories were introduced. The prevalence rate of 0.62 in 100 is reported globally but the Centers for Disease Control and Prevention report it as 1 in 65. Causes are associated with genetic, neurobiological and environmental links. Conditions associated with ASD include learning disabilities, epilepsy, depression and autism-related catatonia. Teaching and learning interventions for individuals with ASD that are particularly useful for addressing movement programmes include: TEACCH, ABA, PECS, PRT and MDT. All of the interventions outlined have some positive outcomes for children and adults with ASD. Structure, repetition, choice and reinforcement are aspects of all programmes, and are avenues to address the theories of mind blindness, weak central coherence, and the absence of high levels of control and attention. It is also important to consider the learning styles of each individual with ASD and indeed if there are other co-occurring disabilities or conditions present, before deciding on any one intervention.

Introduction to Fundamental Movement Skills

Chapter 2 explores the basic principles and practice of fundamental movement skill (FMS) development from a general perspective. This includes definition, phases, classification of skills, age emergent profiles and approaches to addressing skill development for all. An outline of observation, programme planning and delivery is also provided. The importance of the use of demonstration and feedback to facilitate learning is explored. Open and closed motor skills are explained. The chapter also introduces an understanding of domains of learning. The chapter closes with an outline of what constitutes different mature fundamental movement skills.

Understanding concepts in the world of FMS

This section presents some key definitions and an overview of FMS development.

Motor development is the study of the changes in human behaviour over the lifespan, the processes that underlie these changes and the factors that affect those (Payne and Isaacs, 2011). Scholars of motor development endeavour to find out how the changes in movement occur and to identify factors that influence these changes. Figure 2.1, taken from Gallahue and Ozmun (2006), depicts the process of the phases of motor development across the lifespan.

This section includes:

- Reflexive phase

- Rudimentary phase

- Fundamental phase

- Specialised phase

- Lifelong utilisation

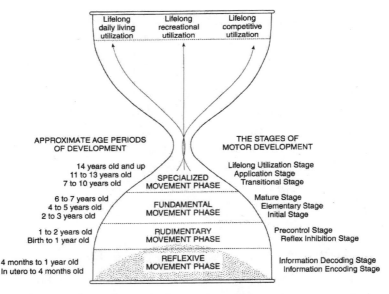

Figure 2.1 Phases of motor development (© Gallahue and Ozmun, 2006).

The reflexive movement phase begins *in utero*, where information encoding and decoding take place. This evolves to the rudimentary movement phase from birth onwards. This includes the inhibition of reflexes present at birth and evolves to the precontrol stage by 1 to 2 years of age. As babies grow and develop in this phase, they sit, grasp, stand and walk alone.

The fundamental movement phase typically develops from 2 years. Fundamental movement skills refer to those skills of movement used in everyday life and these essentially provide the skills necessary to participate in physical activity, games and sports, that is, running, catching, jumping, dodging. These begin to emerge at approximately 2–3 years of age. For each skill, an individual moves through a series of developmental stages, namely initial, elementary and mature.

The initial stage (2–3 years approximately) represents the onset of movement patterns with poor control; parts of the movement sequence are missing and rhythm and coordination are lacking. In the elementary stage (4–5 years approximately) more parts of the sequence are present, with better rhythm and coordination beginning to show. In the mature stage (5–7 years approximately) all movement parts are present, good rhythm and coordination are evident, and movement is mechanically efficient. All children have the potential to be developed in most of the FMS by about 6 years of age. Hand–eye and foot–eye coordination are usually a year or two later. However, these do not develop automatically (naturally). Between-individual differences indicate that the rate of development in skills varies between individuals. Between-skill differences occur when a child may be at mature levels in some skills and may be at initial or elementary levels in others. Within-skill differences are when a child may be at mature stage in leg action of a skill while at elementary level in upper body action. FMS can also be classified as: locomotor, for example, running, hopping, skipping; or manipulation, for example, involving an object such as catching, throwing or balance, which can be either static – standing still – or dynamic – for example, moving and balancing such as in a forward roll.

The specialised phase evolves with refinement and practice through the transitional stage at 7–10 years of age, application at 11–13 years old and lifelong utilisation stages from the age of 14 years upwards.

Lifelong daily living, recreational and competitive utilisation of movement skills are the long-term goals.

KEY POINTS

* Reflexive phase: from the womb to the end of the first year when reflexes disappear.

* Rudimentary phase: babies sit, grasp, stand and walk from 1–2 years.

* Fundamental phase: initial, elementary and mature phases from 2–7 years, where skill development becomes more refined.

* Between-individual differences emerge, i.e. skill development varies with each learner.

* Within-skill differences: may be mature at leg action but elementary at arm action.

* FMS classification: locomotor, manipulation and balance.

* Specialised phase where the learner transitions, applies skills and utilises them.

* Lifelong daily living, recreation and competitive application of skills are the goals.

Why is the development of FMS so important?

This section includes:

* Research on the importance of FMS

* Physical literacy

* ABCs of movement

* Physical activity participation

- Health implications

- Intervention studies

- Skill transfer

FMS are essentially the vocabulary of movement and the kernel of physical literacy. FMS are also believed to be the building blocks for sport-specific skills. They provide us with the ABCs, that is, the agility, balance, coordination and speed necessary for movement. Bellows *et al.* (2017) reported that a motor skill intervention programme in low-income, at-risk pre-schoolers conferred a lasting impact on FMS, specifically object control skills, in these children. Results suggested that at-risk pre-schoolers were already behind in FMS development and these delays were likely to continue through first grade. A longitudinal study by Henrique *et al.* (2016) investigated if baseline motor competence, weight status and sports participation in early childhood predicted sports participation two years later. Results suggested that initial sports participation and more advanced locomotor skills in pre-school years may be important to promote continued participation in sports across childhood. Research has looked at the relationship between FMS development and participation in physical activity among adolescents. Findings established that the higher the competency in FMS, the greater the participation in physical activity (Okely, Booth and Patterson, 2001). In a later study, Okely, Booth and Cheyet (2004) looked at the relationship between body composition and FMS, and found that overweight boys and girls were more likely to possess lower levels of FMS compared to non-overweight participants, that is, those high in FMS proficiency were less likely to be overweight. Lubans *et al.* (2010) carried out a review of associated health benefits in relation to FMS skills of children and adolescents, and established strong evidence for a positive association between FMS and physical activity, that is, those high in FMS competency were more likely to participate in physical activity compared to those who had low proficiency. There was also a positive relationship between FMS competency and cardiorespiratory fitness. A systematic review by Cattuzzo *et al.* (2016) reported that the development of motor competence in childhood may both directly and indirectly augment health-related physical fitness and may serve to enhance the development of long-term health outcomes in children and adolescents. In a 2017 study, Bardid *et al.* examined the effectiveness of a 30-week fundamental motor skill programme in typically developing young children and investigated possible sex differences. The study demonstrated the effectiveness of a wide-scale community-based intervention in typically developing children. The researchers considered that the sex differences reported may indicate the need to use different pedagogical and instructional strategies to enable boys and girls to develop and master a wide range of motor skills. Intervention studies for adolescents and teenagers have also established that improved FMS led to increased participation in physical activity (Ericsson, 2011; Kalaja *et al.*, 2012). Equally the New South Wales Department of Education and Training (2000) indicated that children with proficiency in FMS were found to have greater self-esteem and socialisation skills, which had a knock on effect on other areas of a child's education.

A longitudinal study conducted over seven years by Barnett *et al.* (2009) in New South Wales found that adolescent time spent in moderate-to-vigorous physical activity was positively associated with childhood FMS and, in particular, object control proficiency (kick, catch, throw). The researchers also concluded that object control skills, rather than locomotor skills, appear to be more crucial to total activity time and to activity at higher intensity. Research evidence also exists for successful interventions for post-primary school children and adults, where skills were acquired over time and demonstrated transferability with appropriate practice; Rose and Heath (1990) taught adults (18–22 years) how to throw prior to teaching a tennis serve. Those who learnt to throw learnt to serve more quickly and more easily. Similarly, O'Keeffe *et al.* (2007) taught throwing to teenagers (15.8 years). These researchers concluded that being able to throw facilitated learning of a badminton overhead clear and also transferred to javelin throwing.

KEY POINTS

* Research on the importance of FMS: introduces key studies.

* Physical literacy: provides the alphabet of movement.

* ABCs of movement: agility, balance, coordination and speed.

* Physical activity participation: acquiring FMS promotes participation in physical activity.

* Health implications: acquiring FMS is positively associated with reduced incidences of obesity and cardiovascular disease, high self-esteem and improved social skills.

* Intervention studies: intervening with FMS programmes is successful in developing skills.

* Skill transfer: skills are transferrable to different sports.

How are FMS developed?

FMS do not occur naturally but need to be taught and accompanied by appropriate opportunities to practise and refine them. According to Gallahue and Ozmun (2006), activities addressing FMS acquisition need to be developmentally appropriate. Visual demonstrations need to be provided for each skill being taught and appropriate equipment needs to be used. Clear instruction and feedback are essential for progress in skill acquisition. Learners need opportunities to generalise skills and equally need to be challenged, as well as encouraged, in a safe and positive learning environment.

This section includes:

- The factors that contribute to FMS development

- The facilitation of development from initial stages to mature stages of FMS

What are the factors that contribute to FMS development?

Identified factors that contribute to FMS development include growth, maturation, learning in general and specifically motor learning. Growth refers to quantitative body changes, that is, changes in size of bones, muscles, nervous systems and organs. These changes influence how we move. Maturation (process of ripening) refers to qualitative changes, for example, bone ossification, hormonal changes at puberty and functional changes in the way we move (e.g. mature stage in stages of development). General learning considers changes in behaviour as a consequence of practice or experience, while motor learning specifically considers changes in how we move as a result of practice.

The facilitation of development from initial stages to mature stages of FMS

There is still some misunderstanding regarding the necessity for teaching and learning of FMS. Children do not develop FMS automatically, contrary to popular belief.

> Children do not develop FMS naturally through maturational processes. These skills need to be learned, practised and reinforced. (Logan et al., 2011, p.1)

Unfortunately, many still have the notion that children somehow 'automatically' learn how to perform these fundamental movements. (Gallahue and Ozmun, 2006, p.56)

Some child development experts (not in the motor development area) have written repeatedly about the 'natural' unfolding of the child's movement and play skills and the idea that children develop these abilities merely by growing older. (Gallahue and Ozmun, 2002, p.49)

Teachers, coaches, health practitioners and parents have to consciously work to make children more skilful, and equally they themselves must know how to achieve this. A variety and combination of teaching styles can be used to promote learning. Facilitators must know the component parts and key factors of skills and also be able to identify stages of development for each of the components. They must also know how to correct and improve skills, and the appropriate tasks and practices to set in this regard.

KEY POINTS

* The factors that contribute to FMS development: these include body growth and maturation, learning in general and specifically motor learning, where changes in movement occur as a result of practice.

* The facilitation of development from initial stages to mature stages of FMS: skills need to be learnt, practised and reinforced.

Observation of FMS

This section includes:

* Benefits of observation

* Effective observation

Observation of participants completing FMS provides essential information for programme planning. Observation also gives the opportunity to provide students with feedback and to evaluate the effectiveness of a teaching and learning session. So what are key aspects of effective observation? Observation should occur in a natural setting without informing students they are being observed. The facilitator should consider how the movement actually looks rather than focusing on the actual outcome of the movement. Observation should always be objective and ideally involve more than one facilitator. As skills need to be generalised to a number of different contexts, so too should observation of these skills.

KEY POINTS

* Purpose of observation: provide information for programme planning, evaluation and learner feedback.

* Effective observation: should take place in natural settings.

* Focus on how the movement looks.

* Generalise observation to different contexts.

Programme planning of FMS

This section includes:

* When to start FMS

* How long to acquire FMS

* How many FMS skills to teach together

* Session planning

* Environmental factors

Planning for the development of FMS should start as early as possible in a child's overall school programme. According to the New South Wales Department of Education and Training (2000) 240–600 minutes of actual instruction time are necessary to develop an FMS to proficiency. They also recommend focusing on just four skills per year to try and ensure proficiency is attained. This of course is contingent on students being provided with opportunity to practise each of the skills. Addressing FMS development and attainment should adopt both a bottom-up and a top-down approach especially in educational settings. Similarly, in therapeutic settings it is important that all disciplines work together and ensure parents are active collaborators in each FMS programme. Each FMS session should include an introduction, a teaching component and a practising component. The introduction should include a warm up where, when ready, students can work in small groups and reinforce previously acquired knowledge of the skill. When teaching a skill, the skill should be clearly demonstrated with consistent teaching cues, appropriate feedback and technique correction, and include questions to explore students' learning of the skill components. Practising of the skill should happen both individually and in small groups, with the skill also incorporated into simple games, focusing on teaching specific components and using a variety of equipment. Organising and managing the environment is essential to the successful delivery of FMS programmes. Working indoors provides clear boundaries, space is possibly limited, observation of participants is well controlled and verbal cues are more easily taken on board. When outdoors the boundaries are less controlled, resources need to be organised beforehand and environmental conditions can be changeable. This means verbal instructions may need to be adapted and non-verbal cues included.

KEY POINTS

* When to start FMS: as early in primary school as possible.

* How long to acquire FMS: 240–600 minutes per skill to proficiency.

* How many FMS skills to teach: focus on four per year.

* Session planning: include introduction with stretches, teaching and practice components.

* Teaching a skill: include demonstration, cues, feedback, correction, practice, and question and answer session.

* Environmental factors: plan resources for both indoor and outdoor sessions.

Delivering an FMS programme

This section includes:

* FMS instruction

* Role of facilitator

When delivering FMS instruction to participants at the initial and elementary levels of development the entire skill needs to be introduced. The skill should be clearly demonstrated followed by an opportunity for the participant to explore it. New skills can be compared with similar skills and contextualised to different activities. Feedback should be immediate and precise without focusing on the product of the performance. For participants moving towards mature patterns of a skill, providing opportunities to practise in a variety of settings is essential. It is equally important to simulate practice sessions to mimic real-life individual or game situations. Appropriate instruction, checking for understanding, and providing demonstrations and feedback are essential. Facilitators need to be correctly positioned, start/stop signals should be consistent (e.g. a whistle), distractions should be at a minimum and participants should be engaged with succinct instructions. Verbal cues should also be consistent, should be short and simple, and closely aligned with the actual demonstration of the skill. Facilitators should check for the participants' understanding of the skill by checking if the participants are able to recall or demonstrate what was learnt. Use of demonstration and feedback is dealt with in detail in the next sections.

KEY POINTS

* FMS instruction: introduce the whole skill with demonstration and practice.

* Role of facilitator: provide instruction, demonstration, feedback and check for understanding.

Use of demonstration to facilitate the learning of FMS

This section includes:

- Rationale for demonstration

- When is it used

- Cognitive mediation theory

- Role of the facilitator

Learners can be given information directly through instruction and demonstration (command style of teaching) or they can create (construct) their own information and knowledge (discovery style of teaching). Effective teaching and learning can be brought about by a combination of teaching styles and methods. With appropriate use of demonstration, learners can both receive and construct knowledge about the skill being learnt. Learning from demonstration involves both perceiving behaviour and then imitating it, which we seem to be neurologically wired to do. So when is demonstration actually used to best effect? Demonstration is used when we are teaching a 'new' movement pattern for a skill (coordination) and when there are 'new' tactics or a pattern of play, for example, organisation of where to go, who to pass to, etc. Demonstration is also used in a lesson or practice in which a 'new' drill is to be performed or a 'new' game to be played. Demonstration gives information about 'What to do?' in the cognitive stage of learning (Fitts and Posner, 1967) and facilitates getting 'the idea of the movement' (Gentile's 1972/2000 model).

Cognitive mediation theory is used to explain how demonstrations work (Bandura, 1986). The learner transforms information by means of cognitive (mental) processes into memory, which then serves to guide future behaviour. The cognitive processes involved are attention, retention, reproduction and motivation. Facilitators can use Bandura's theory as a guide to set up a demonstration and facilitate the cognitive learning processes. It can also act as a tool for diagnosis and correction as participants attempt the skill being learnt. To facilitate attention, it is important to consider positioning, the distance and the angles involved. In relation to positioning, participants should have their backs to another class or an ongoing activity and indeed to the sun so they can engage undistracted. Distance needs to be considered because if participants are too close, they cannot see. Equally, the whole notion of angles being taken into account is essential, as, in the case of large groups, those on the sides have a different view from those in the middle, so it is important to demonstrate from different angles. To facilitate retention, the skill needs to be repeated a number of times and once again from different angles.

Reproduction is all about 'having a go'. Here it's important to consider the facilitator behaviour when the participant is having a go. First, the facilitator needs to stand back and observe (on the periphery), allow participants to explore, make errors as part of the learning process and understand that participants are constructing their own knowledge about the skill (constructivist theory). The facilitator should consider whether the learners are self-correcting and know what to look for in relation to the key factors and the teaching points of the skill. As the session progresses, the facilitator should note if the class in general has got the idea of the movement and, if necessary, demonstrate again and emphasise a particular point. If there is any participant who needs help, it should be given at this point. In relation to positioning, when giving corrective feedback, the facilitator should be able to see the whole class, give a word of encouragement to someone at the other end or note other pupils who need help.

Using Bandura's cognitive processes helps the facilitator to analyse and diagnose the source of problems. This may be during attention or retention. Often, because of a lack of attention, the participant may not know, understand or remember what they are trying do. The facilitator should be able to identify this and re-explain and demonstrate again. If the problem is one of reproduction (coordination), the facilitator can give corrective feedback, which makes the task easier (adaptation). In relation to the amount and frequency of demonstration, the facilitator should demonstrate sufficiently before the initial attempt, to prepare learners to 'have a go' and then repeat intermittently as needed. Demonstration using both video and sound has been found to be effective in enhancing the learning of a skill at this stage. Motivation emerges with both feedback and success (See next section).

KEY POINTS

* Rationale for demonstration: learners can receive and construct knowledge of a skill.

- When is it used: used for new movement patterns, new tactics and new games.

- Cognitive mediation theory: consists of attention, retention, reproduction and motivation.

- Role of the facilitator: consider positioning, encourage 'having a go', adapting as necessary and motivating.

Use of feedback to facilitate the learning of FMS

This section includes:

- Intrinsic feedback

- Extrinsic feedback

- When to give feedback

- How to give feedback

When a person performs a skill they have available to them feedback information that tells them about: (a) the outcome of the skill (did they achieve what they intended to achieve?), and (b) how they performed the skill (Magill, 2011). They also get feedback from the teacher/coach/facilitator. Feedback can be intrinsic or extrinsic. Intrinsic feedback is made up of internal and external feedback, which includes visual, auditory, proprioceptive and tactile systems. Proprioception is an awareness of the position of any body part in space, and of the relation of any body part to the rest of the body. Proprioceptive information is essential to the normal functioning of the body's mechanical control system, and is normally acquired unconsciously from sense receptors in the muscles, joints, tendons and the balance organ of the inner ear. Extrinsic feedback comes from the facilitator, teacher or coach. Extrinsic feedback provides the participant with knowledge of results and knowledge of performance. Intrinsic feedback in practice provides information to the participant as a natural consequence of the execution of a skill. An experienced performer makes use of this feedback (particularly proprioceptive and tactile) to take corrective action during the skill or on the next attempt or indeed to adjust the next part of a movement plan. However, a beginner is not in a position to interpret intrinsic feedback or know what corrective action to take based on it. Augmented feedback from the teacher or coach can enable the learning of how to interpret intrinsic feedback. For the novice learner, initially proprioceptive (internal, kinaesthetic) feedback is often meaningless. Good use of teacher and coach feedback can help the learner to make sense of and use of proprioceptive (kinaesthetic) feedback by getting them to focus on the 'feel' of the skill. Equally, feedback should be corrective and motivational and give information about the key factors of a skill. In relation to the frequency of feedback, the facilitator should start with more frequent feedback and withdraw as the skill evolves to prevent dependency. Receiving information about errors that leads to improvements in performance is motivational. It leads to greater competency by the learner and encourages them to keep trying to improve. How the facilitator gives feedback makes a difference to motivation and confidence (self-efficacy) and to what the learner can achieve (Mouratidis, Lens and Vansteenkiste, 2010). Studies by Lewthwaite and Wulf (2010) and Avila *et al.* (2012) show that positive feedback in addition to information feedback (about error and correction) lead to better learning. Motivation, self-efficacy and perceived competence are also increased compared to just receiving information.

KEY POINTS

* Intrinsic feedback: is internal and external feedback, which includes visual, auditory, proprioceptive and tactile systems.

* Proprioception: is an awareness of the position of any body part in space, and of the relation of any body part to the rest of the body.

* Extrinsic feedback: comes from the facilitator, teacher or coach.

* When to give feedback: the facilitator should start with more frequent feedback and withdraw as the skill evolves.

* How to give feedback: feedback should be corrective and motivational and give information about the key factors of a skill.

Understanding closed and open motor skills

This section includes:

* What are motor skills

* Classification of motor skills

* Stability of the environment

* Gentile's teaching guide

* Teaching games for understanding

A motor skill is defined by Magill (1993) as 'an action or a task that has a goal and that requires voluntary body and/or limb movement to achieve the goal' (p.7). Motor skills are often classified according to what aspects of each skill are common to another. However, motor skills do not necessarily have to fit into any one category exclusively. Common classification systems include the precision of movement involved in the skills, defining beginning and end points and considering the stability of the environment. These are further broken down as follows: the precision of movement category involves both gross and fine motor skills. Gross motor skills include using the large muscles of the body in a coordinated movement pattern, for example, jumping, running. Fine motor skills involve using the small muscles of the body with a high degree of precision, for example, writing, fastening a button. This classification is typically used in rehabilitative and special education settings. Defining beginning and end points considers when a skill begins and ends. Subcategories include discrete, serial and continuous motor skills. Discrete motor skills have beginning and end points defined by an object being moved or altered, for example, picking up a pen. A serial motor skill involves putting a number of discrete skills together in a series, for example, writing a letter, which includes picking up the aforementioned pen. Continuous motor skills are those skills that involve the performer repeating the movement during the performance of the skill and beginning and end points are hence dictated by the performer, for example, running.

The stability of the environment considers whether the environment is changing or not. The subcategories here include closed and open motor skills. Closed skills include any skill that takes place in a stable and unchanging environment, for example, climbing up stairs. Open motor skills on the other hand take place in a changing environment where the participant must act according to the action of the object or the environment, that is, when catching a ball in a game the player must move as dictated by the direction/trajectory of the ball.

Gentile's (1972/2000) teaching model is used as a guide for appropriate teaching and practice for closed and open skills. The model has two key goals. The goal of stage one is to get the idea of the movement and to distinguish between regulatory (relevant) and non-regulatory (non-relevant) stimuli (information). There is no distinction in stage one between closed and open skills. The goal of stage two is that of fixation and diversification and there are definite closed and open skill differences. In relation to closed skills in stage two, the learners are encouraged to practise in a stable, predictable environment to stabilise the action pattern. They should know what to focus attention on and practise that focus. Simulation practice is developed when a pattern becomes stable. Distractions are built in to gradually simulate the competitive context, for example, rebounders, crowd noise, being out of breath or fatigued and having being involved in previous play. A common fault is not to have appropriate practice. Hence practice must be structured to maximise the transfer from the practice context to the competitive context. In relation to open skills, learners are provided with the opportunity to initially get the idea of the movement in a stable environment, that is, the same as with closed skills. They are encouraged to practise variations of the basic pattern of the movement skill. Gradually this is moved to a more dynamic context where variations in the action pattern, opponents and decision-making are included. At this stage, the space of the practice area should also be reduced. When teaching a closed skill, the facilitator should begin with a closed environment and gradually move to an open environment. The facilitator teaches the learners to look and see (Where are team mates and opponents? Who is free? Who is moving into the free space?). At this stage, errors are corrected using re-enactment. Gentile's model implies the use of the direct/command style of teaching. However, basic movement patterns can be acquired using discovery (indirect) methods too.

In the case of games, FMS may be taught through the 'games for understanding' method, whereby the concept of the game is acquired before learning and refining the specific skills. In all cases, however, the teacher needs to know: (a) the key factors in order to be able to guide and correct learners, and (b) where participants/performers need to direct their attention. This is in order to obtain information for effective performance and, in the case of games, make correct decisions.

KEY POINTS

* What are motor skills: defined by Magill as 'an action or a task that has a goal and that requires voluntary body and/or limb movement to achieve the goal'.

* Classification of motor skills: can be fine (involve small muscles, e.g. fingers) or gross (involve large muscles, e.g. legs).

- Motor skills can also be: discrete motor skills (have beginning and end points defined by an object being moved), serial motor skills (involves putting a number of discrete skills together in a series) and continuous motor skills (involve the performer repeating the movement during the performance of the skill).

- Stability of the environment: closed skills include any skill that takes place in a stable and unchanging environment. Open motor skills on the other hand take place in a changing environment.

- Gentile's teaching model, stage one: the goal of stage one is to get the idea of the movement and to distinguish between regulatory (relevant) and non-regulatory (non-relevant) stimuli (information). In this stage there is no distinction between closed and open skills.

- Gentile's teaching model, stage two: the goal of stage two is that of fixation and diversification.

- Definite closed differences: practise in a stable, predictable environment.

- Open skill differences: this is moved to a more dynamic context where variations in the action pattern, opponents and decision-making are included.

- Teaching games for understanding: learn the skills in a games context.

Understanding domains of learning

This section includes:

- Domains of learning

- Practice

- Fitts and Posner

- Bernstein's degrees of freedom

Bloom *et al.* (1956) identified three key domains as areas to be developed by education curricula. These included cognitive, affective/social and psychomotor domains. Payne and Isaac (2002) added the fourth physical domain. The cognitive domain includes intellectual development (ideas, ways of thinking and reasoning). The affective/social domain looks at the development of social interaction and feelings of self-worth grown with responses from others. The psychomotor domain is the domain of movement development. The physical domain encompasses changes in anatomical and physiological systems. The psychomotor domain is often the one that gets the least attention due to lack of emphasis on physical education in school settings. All of these domains undergo age-related change and act and develop in an interactive way. An example of this interaction can be seen as follows: an infant is creeping towards an object (stimulus) and developing gross motor skills (psychomotor domain). Muscles are challenged (physical) and a beginning knowledge of space and distance is emerging (cognitive domain). The child grasps and manipulates the object developing fine motor skills (psychomotor domain) and develops knowledge about the object (cognitive domain). With approval from parents, the child gets a sense of achievement and feeling of self-worth (affective domain). From the learning to move, moving to learn philosophy we know that cognitive and affective learning is important, but, as Gallahue and Donnelly (2003, p.248) indicate, 'it is equally important for children to become skilful movers'.

Everyone, including the greatest of champions, has to learn as beginners and is still learning as long as they wish to improve. Learning is the process of acquiring a skill and occurs through practice. Performance is the execution of the skill. Practice is repeated performance (attempted performance) of a skill. When can a skill be said to be learnt? The limits are not really known. The criteria include (a) when the basic movement pattern is acquired and can be performed consistently; (b) when the perfect score is obtained or 50 per cent or 75 per cent, etc.; or (c) when the learner reaches a proficiency level to enable them to participate/play with peers with enjoyment. As a skill improves there is often less return for a lot of practice, but very small improvements are significant. Competitions are won, points are scored etc. by fractions of a second and centimetres. Practice distinguishes experts (highly skilled) from non-experts (low skilled). Research shows that an essential distinguishing feature between experts in a wide variety of fields (e.g. sports champions, top class musicians and dancers) and those who are not experts is the amount of practice over many years (Ericsson et al., 1993; Ericsson, 2011; Starkes et al., 1996). The concept of deliberate practice is thousands of hours of practice over a number of years. In the Fitts and Posner (1967) model of learning, the beginner is in the thinking stage of learning during practice, the intermediate learner is in the doing/practice stage and the advanced learner is in the automatic stage. The beginner is asking, 'what do I do?' The intermediate learner has less thinking, less or no self-talk, less attention demanding, movements are seen more in wholes, completion of one part is associated with the beginning of the next part and the development of an associated feel (kinaesthetic/proprioceptive) for the movement. For the advanced learner, there is little or no thinking/attention needed, skill is automatic and permanent, and the mind free to focus on what is happening in the surrounding environment for decision-making.

Bernstein's model of motor learning introduced the notion of degrees of freedom in relation to learning. For the first stage the learner is in the coordination stage and needs to take control over their degrees of freedom. Freezing of degrees of freedom is a strategy employed by beginners to simplify and create temporary workable patterns. In stage two the learner is in the control stage and freeing of the degrees of freedom occurs. When this happens, degrees of freedom are linked appropriately to each other to act as functional units, for example, shoulder–elbow–wrist and hip–knee–ankle. Each joint is activated at the appropriate time. Stage three is the exploitation (dexterity) skill stage, with a stable but adaptable movement pattern. The learner is able to make moment-to-moment adjustments to ever-changing environmental conditions. In relation to the Bernstein (1967) model, the focus is on changes in movement patterns with practice and learning. With the Fitts and Posner (1967) model, the focus is on changes in thinking with practice and learning. The learner is moving from conscious thinking and attention to automatic thinking and attention. Continuums exist in each model. Having knowledge of these models lets the facilitator know how learning occurs and they are in a better position to know how to facilitate it. Equally, knowing about difficulties learners have can make facilitators more understanding of learners. The facilitator can modify constraints, adapt decision-making strategies and assess learning in different ways.

KEY POINTS

* Domains of learning: four key domains of learning include cognitive, affective, psychomotor and physical.

* Practice: one of the distinguishing features of experts is the amount they practise over the years.

* Fitts and Posner's model: focus is on changes in thinking with practice and learning.

* Bernstein's model: focus is on changes in movement patterns with practice and learning.

Assessment of FMS development

Assessment of fundamental movement skill development provides much-needed information on whether participants are learning the skills in order to evaluate effectiveness of the programme. Strategies to assess FMS development can include observation, skills tests, assessment of performance, rating scales, peer assessment, self-assessment and anecdotal feedback, or a combination of all of these. Regardless of which strategy is used, all assessments should engage the participants. Assessments should be clear, recognise achievement and be manageable. Participant portfolios that contain all information including audio, video and written content are a useful way of managing files for each individual. Assessment is explored further in Chapter 4.

Mature FMS

The next section includes a selection of FMS with visual support, voiceover prompts and identifying features for each skill. The www.getautismactive.com website provides video demonstrations of these skills in action. Identifying features are included, which provide a list of key components of each skill when broken down. In the sample workbook provided here and on the www.getautismactive.com website, there is also a section to add comments and reflect on how a skill is developing or a programme is going. Equally, on the website there is a video demonstration of each skill being taught. These videos provide the facilitator and the learner with a better understanding of each individual skill and its component parts. To further enhance and develop the acquisition of knowledge regarding fundamental movement skills, it is recommended that facilitators from disciplines come together in communities of practice (Crawford, O'Reilly and Flanagan, 2012). These sessions can include both theoretical and practical components. Equally it is useful for facilitators to look at videos of participants at different stages of skill development.

Skills included are presented as follows:

- balance on a balance beam
- ball bouncing
- ball rolling
- catching
- dodging
- forward roll
- hitting a ball with a bat
- hopping
- horizontal jump
- jumping from a height
- kicking
- leaping
- overarm throw
- running
- skipping
- sliding
- static balance
- vertical jump
- volleying.

Balance on a balance beam
Voiceover instructions

– Keep head up.

- Use alternate steps.

- Use the arms at will.

Identifying features

- Can walk a balance beam.

- Alternate stepping action is used.

- The eyes focus beyond the stepper.

- Both arms are used to aid balance.

Ball bouncing
Voiceover instructions

- Push the ball.

- Use your fingertips.

- Follow through.

Identifying features

- Feet are placed in narrow strike position, with opposite foot forward.

- Slight forward trunk lean/leaning slightly forward.

- Ball is held waist high.

- Ball is pushed towards the ground, with follow-through of arm, wrist and fingers.

- There is controlled force of downward thrust.

- Repeated contact and pushing action is initiated from the fingertips.
- Visual monitoring is unnecessary/no need to watch the ball.
- Controlled dribbling occurs.

Ball rolling
Voiceover instructions

- Keep your eyes on the target.
- Keep the knees bent.
- Roll the ball off your fingers.
- Transfer weight from back to front foot.

Identifying features

- Stride stance is present/legs are apart.
- Slight hip rotation and trunk lean forward/lean slightly forward.
- Pronounced knee bend is present.
- There is forward swing, with weight transferred from rear to forward foot/when swinging forward with the ball, the weight is transferred to the front foot.
- The ball is released at knee level or below.
- Eyes are on the target throughout.

Catching
Voiceover instructions

- Keep your eyes on the ball.

- Reach for the ball.

- Let the arms give on contact/let the arms relax on contact.

- Keep hands on the sides of the ball.

Identifying features

- There is no avoidance reaction/the head does not turn away.

- Eyes follow the ball into the hands.

- Arms are held relaxed at the sides, and forearms are held in front of body.

- Arms give on contact to absorb the force of the ball.

- Arms adjust to the flight of the ball.

- Thumbs are held in opposition to each other/thumbs are held opposite to each other.

- Hands grasp the ball in a well-timed, simultaneous motion.

- Fingers grasp more effectively.

▓ Dodging
Voiceover instructions

- Keep the knees bent.

- Put the lead foot down hard and push off/put the front foot down hard and push off.

- Run at the target.

- Fake.

- Push off in the other direction.

Identifying features

- Knees bent, a slight trunk lean forward.

- Fluid directional changes, performs well in all directions.

- Head and shoulders fake/move head and shoulders in the other direction.

- Good lateral movement.

Forward roll
Voiceover instructions

- Curl up.

- Push off hard.

- Keep the body in a tight 'c' shape.

- Return to a standing position.

Identifying features

- Head leads the action.

- Back of the head touches surface lightly.

- Body remains in tight 'c'.

- Arms aid in force production.

- Momentum returns student to starting position.

Hopping
Voiceover instructions

- Raise the thigh of your hopping leg until it's parallel to the ground.

— Use your arms alternately.

Identifying features

— Non-support leg is flexed at 90 degrees or less.

— Body lean is present/slight lean forward.

— There is swinging action of the non-support leg.

— Arms move rhythmically.

— Arms are used for force production.

Horizontal jump
Voiceover instructions

— Crouch down.

— Swing your arms backwards and then forwards.

— Tip the trunk forward.

— Stretch and reach forward.

— Rotate forward and up to a standing position.

— Ensure the heels contact the ground first on landing.

— Give on landing.

Identifying features

— Arms move high and to the rear during preparatory crouch.

— During take-off, the arms swing forward with force and reach high.

— Arms are held high throughout jumping action.

- Trunk is propelled at approximately 45 degree angle.

- There is major emphasis on horizontal distance.

- Engage a deep preparatory crouch.

- Ensure complete extension at take-off.

- Thighs are held parallel to the ground during flight; lower leg lands vertically.

- Body weight is forward at landing.

Jumping from a height
Voiceover instructions

- Lean forward slightly.

- Move your arms forward or sideways.

- Keep your legs shoulder width apart.

- Give at the knees when landing.

- Land on the balls of the feet.

Identifying features

- Ensure two-footed take-off.

- Have a controlled flight phase.

- Both arms are used to control balance as needed.

- Feet contact the lower surface simultaneously, with toes touching first.

- Feet land shoulder width apart.

- Flexion occurs at the knees and hip.

▓ Kicking

Voiceover instructions

- Keep your eyes on the ball.

- Stand behind the ball and slightly to one side.

- Step forward on your non-kicking foot.

- Swing your kicking leg back and forward with force.

- Contact the ball with the instep of the foot.

- Follow through in the direction of the target.

- Use your arms for balance.

Identifying features

- Arms swing in opposition to each other during kicking action.

- Trunk bends at the waist during follow-through.

- Movement of kicking leg is initiated at the hip.

- Support leg bends slightly on contact.

- Length of leg swing increases.

- Follow-through is high.

- Approach to the ball is from either a run or leap.

▓ Leaping

Voiceover instructions

- Push upward and forward with your back foot.

- Stretch and reach with your forward foot.

- Keep the head up and lean forward.
- Use alternate arm and leg action.

Identifying features

- Ensure relaxed rhythmical action.
- Have forceful extension of take-off leg.
- Have a definite forward trunk lean.
- Ensure definite arm opposition.
- Have full extension of legs during flight.

Overarm throw
Voiceover instructions

- Turn to the side.
- Swing arm backwards.
- Let the throwing elbow move forward.
- Take a long step forward with the opposite leg.

Identifying features

- Arm is swung backwards in preparation.
- Opposite elbow is raised for balance.
- Throwing elbow moves forward horizontally as it extends.
- Trunk markedly rotates to throwing side during preparatory action.
- Throwing shoulder drops slightly.

- Definite rotation occurs through hips, legs, spine and shoulders during throw.

- Weight during preparatory movement is on the rear foot.

- As weight is shifted, there is a step with the opposite foot.

Running
Voiceover instructions

- Keep your head up.

- Lean slightly into run.

- Use your arms alternately.

- Lift your knees.

- Run lightly.

Identifying features

- Stride length is at maximum.

- Speed is fast.

- Ensure a definite flight phase.

- Ensure extension of the support leg.

- Recovery thigh should be parallel to the ground.

- Arms swing vertically in opposition to the legs.

Skipping
Voiceover instructions

- Step forward and hop on the same foot.

- Repeat with the other foot.

- Lift knees upwards.

- Swing your arms upwards with your legs.

Identifying features

- Rhythmical weight transfer is present throughout.

- Rhythmical use of arms occurs throughout.

- Ensure low vertical lift on hop.

- Toe is first on landing.

▨ Sliding
Voiceover instructions

- Step to the side and draw the second foot quickly to the first foot.

- Repeat the action.

- Use your arms.

- Move on the balls of your feet.

- Bend the knees slightly.

Identifying features

- Smooth, rhythmical action is maintained.

- Trailing leg lands adjacent to or behind the lead leg.

- There is a low flight pattern.

- Heel–toe contact combination occurs.

- Arms are not needed for balance.

▨ Static balance
Voiceover instructions

- Hold your arms out to the side.

- Focus on an object.

Identifying features

- Balances with eyes closed.

- Uses arms and trunk as needed.

- Lifts non-supporting leg.

- Focuses on the non-dominant leg.

▨ Hitting a ball with a bat
Voiceover instructions

- Ensure your hands are touching when holding the bat.

- Keep your eyes on the ball.

- Swing back and then forward.

- Contact the ball when the arm is straight.

- Follow through to the chest.

Identifying features

- Trunk turns to the side in anticipation of the tossed ball.

- Weight shifts to the back foot.

- Hips rotate.

- Weight shifts to the forward foot, which occurs while the object is approaching.
- Striking occurs in a long, full arc in a horizontal pattern.
- Weight shifts to forward foot at contact.

Vertical jump
Voiceover instructions

- Crouch down for take-off.
- Jump explosively upwards.
- Swing your arms upwards.
- Stretch and look upwards.
- Extend your reaching arm at the shoulder.

Identifying features

- Preparatory crouch with knee flexion.
- Forceful extension occurs at the hips, knees and ankles.
- Simultaneous coordinated upward arm lift is present.
- There is upward head tilt with eyes focused on the target.
- Full body extension occurs.
- There is elevation of the reaching arm.
- Controlled landing occurs very close to the point of take-off.

Volleying
Voiceover instructions

- Be in position beneath the ball.

- Watch the flight of the ball.

- Extend your arms and legs as the ball contacts your fingers.

- Follow through in the direction of the ball.

Identifying features

- The participant gets under the ball.

- There is good contact with the fingertips.

- The wrists remain stiff and the arms follow through.

- The participant is able to control the direction and intended flight of the ball.

Summary

Chapter 2 explored the principles and practice of FMS from initial to mature stages, providing guidance on how these skills are best acquired. The importance of addressing FMS development was outlined from the benefits of engaging in physical activity and preventing obesity to acquiring sport-specific skills. Growth, maturation and motor learning were identified as factors contributing to the development of FMS. The facilitation of moving from the initial to the mature stages of development was explored, especially considering the role of the facilitator in supporting the use of demonstration, feedback and developing knowledge of closed and open motor skills. Gentile's and Bloom's taxonomy were introduced as was Bernstein's model of degrees of freedom. The chapter closed with an outline of a series of mature FMS including voiceover instructions and identifying features for each particular skill as depicted on the www.getautismactive.com website.

CHAPTER 3

Autism and Fundamental Movement Skill Research

This chapter explores research studies in relation to fundamental movement skills (FMS) and autism spectrum disorder (ASD). In particular studies confirming the presence of motor impairment are considered. Motor skill intervention studies are also explored, as are comparative studies of physical activity levels among children with and without ASD. Studies of this nature are essential and welcome. However, criticism of some of the research includes small sample sizes, lack of consistency of diagnostic criteria among studies, methodology issues with a variety of tools being used and a lack of intervention studies in the field.

Motor impairment and ASD

In relation to movement skills and ASD, Reid and Collier (2002) stated:

> General statements of skill delay or proficiency were best directed at groups of people and should be based on wide evidence, including empirical investigations, case studies and clinical observations. Given the available data, we believe the most appropriate conclusion is that movement skills are often poorly delayed in ASD, individual exceptions notwithstanding. (Reid and Collier, 2002, p.20)

Confirmation of motor impairment for individuals with ASD

This section includes:

- Research confirmation of motor impairment

Movement studies from infancy to adulthood for individuals on the spectrum will now be considered. Teitelbaum *et al.* (1998) identified difficulties in early movement skill behaviours, including lying posture and pattern of crawling in infants (6–12 months) with ASD using retrospective video analysis. Research studies of Flanagan, Perry and Freeman (2012) and Landa (2008) also concurred with the occurrence of motor delay evident in infants with ASD. Lloyd, MacDonald and Lord (2013), examining children at 36 months, found the presence of motor delay increased with increasing age. With a 3- to 4-year-old age group Jasmin *et al.* (2009) found the incidence of motor delay was significant compared to normative data. Liu and Breslin (2013) examined children with ASD aged between 3 and 16 years and found motor delay persistent compared to peers with typical development. The purpose of a study by McDonald *et al.* (2013) was to determine whether the functional motor skills of 6- to 15-year-old children with high functioning ASD predicted success in standardised social communicative skills. A total of 35 children with ASD between the ages of 6 and 15 years participated in this study. Object control motor skills significantly predicted calibrated ASD severity. The researchers concluded that children with weaker motor skills have greater social communicative skill deficits. In a study by Staples and Reid (2010) the motor skill performance of 9- to 12-year-old children with ASD was compared to three groups of typically developing children matched on chronological age, movement skill or cognitive ability. Children with ASD performed similarly on locomotor and object control subtests, demonstrating significant delays relative to their chronological age, with the majority performing similar to children approximately half their age (4–6 years). These movement skill impairments were also greater than would be expected given their cognitive level. Pan, Tsai and Chu (2009) also found significant group differences based on performance of both locomotor and object control skills between 6- to 10-year-old boys with ASD and their typically developing peers of similar age. This study also conducted separate analyses to examine the performance of individual skills and the results demonstrated that children with ASD had particular difficulty with two locomotor (gallop and hop) and four object control (strike, dribble, catch, roll) skills.

An earlier study by Hilton *et al.* (2007) examined the correlation between severity of Asperger's disorder and motor impairment. Children with Asperger's disorder aged 6–12 years of age (n = 51) and a control group of typically developed children also aged 6–12 years (n = 56) were assessed using the Social Responsiveness Scale (SRS) and the Movement Assessment Battery for Children (MABC). Strong correlations were found between the MABC motor impairment scores and the SRS severity levels. The researchers concluded that the degree of correlation indicated that motor skill impairment is a function of severity within SRS for children with Asperger's disorder. In the earlier research of Berkeley *et al.* (2001), the skills of 15 children (10 male, 5 female) with high functioning ASD were compared to national scores, and participants with high functioning ASD were found to have delayed fundamental motor skills compared to national scores. In the research of Manjiviona and Prior (1995), the motor skills of children with high functioning ASD were compared with those of children with Asperger's disorder, and findings indicated that 50 per cent of the children with Asperger's disorder and 66.7 per cent of the children with high functioning ASD had definite motor problems. A comparative examination of 'clumsiness' in ASD, Asperger's disorder and pervasive developmental disorder – not otherwise specified (PDD-NOS) by Ghaziuddin and Butler (1998) found coordination deficits in all three groups. In earlier research, Morin and Reid (1985) examined whether delayed motor development was due to ASD or learning disability, and concluded that delayed motor function in low functioning individuals with ASD might be more reflective of accompanying learning disabilities than ASD, which they indicated was of great concern for practitioners in the field.

In summary, motor problems are clearly common to individuals on the spectrum and have now been identified to be present from infancy and to become progressively more marked with increasing age.

KEY POINT

* Research confirmation of motor impairment: findings over time indicate that motor impairment has been confirmed from infancy to teenage years in ASD.

Motor skill interventions and ASD

This section includes:

* Motor skill intervention effects for participants with ASD

This section examines findings in relation to movement skill interventions for individuals with ASD. Intensity, frequency and type of activity are examined in detail. Ketcheson, Hauck and Ulrich (2016) explored the effects of an early motor skill intervention on motor skills, levels of physical activity and socialisation in young children with ASD. The pilot study involved 20 children with ASD aged 4–6 years. The experimental group (n = 11) participated in an 8-week intervention consisting of motor skills instruction for 4 h/day, 5 days/week. The control group (n = 9) did not receive the intervention. Statistically significant differences were found between groups in all three motor outcomes: locomotor, object control and gross quotient. The authors concluded that the findings shed light on the importance of including motor programming as part of the early intervention services delivered to young children with ASD. A further study that examined the effectiveness of an FMS intervention on motor outcomes, adaptive behaviour and social skills in 4-year-old children with ASD found that the experimental group achieved significant gains in gross motor skills following a 12-week intervention (Bremer, Balogh and Lloyd, 2014). Significant changes were not reported in either social skills or adaptive behaviour. In a similar study by Bremer and Lloyd (2016), children with ASD (aged 3–7 years) participated in an FMS intervention that consisted of two 6-week instructional blocks. Group 1 attended a 12-week FMS intervention for 1 hour per week, while Group 2 acted as a control. Group 2 then attended a 6-week FMS intervention for 2 hours each week (1 hour per day on two separate days). Despite differences in intervention intensity, both groups received 12 hours of direct instruction, and all sessions were the same between the two groups (i.e. the same instruction and content). Improvements in both motor skill proficiency and social skills were reported.

A study by Crawford and Dorney (2011) examined the effects of a community-based, parent-led physical activity programme on the FMS of children with ASD. The programme was run once per week for 2 hours over a 12-week period, with the support of a newly qualified physical education teacher. The programme provided participants with a variety of games-based activities and taster activities of different sports: soccer, rugby, etc. Parents participated in setting up and running the sessions. The FMS of participating children (n = 14) were assessed. Further qualitative data were generated using parental interviews. Changes were indicative of a positive intervention effect. Key themes emerging from parent interviews included parental belief in the benefits of FMS programmes from both skill developments, health-accrued benefits, enhanced social responsiveness and reduced stereotypical behaviours. They also had an overall desire to be included and actively involved in their children's development and progress. Issues of lack of facilities, training and support for parents to encourage meaningful participation and a lack of established physical activity/sports programmes for teenagers with ASD emerged. This study indicated that when parents were given the opportunity to learn and implement skills that improved their child's functioning, increased positive affect, reduced stress and improved self-efficacy occurred. The researchers concluded that parents should be considered partners or collaborators with practitioners in parent education programmes where they help develop goals and programmes along with the facilitators. Results also revealed lower parental stress, higher levels of confidence and more positive parent–child interactions occurred. Parental knowledge about the child's needs, preferences and history provided the best guide to the appropriate approach or any accommodations that needed to be made. Families are important participants in the development and implementation of programmes because they are the most stable and knowledgeable people in the child's life. When parents are collaborators in treatment, they can learn to use techniques such as differential reinforcement of alternative behaviours (DRA; Neidert, Iwata and Dozier, 2005) at home to help their child appropriately express their needs and prevent the occurrence of behaviour problems. In this instance parents were confident to work on FMS with their children, and had reduced fears about increasing the intensity of activities with appropriate training. Parents and other family members can be taught how to incorporate many different treatment techniques and skills into everyday life, in this instance FMS.

Treating children with ASD involves more than individual therapy and should include the family and any others who spend time with the child. By including families in treatment, the child's prognosis improves as do other factors that are critical to providing a successful treatment (Simpson, 2001).

The research of Crawford, MacDonncha and Smyth (2013) examined the effects of individualised adapted physical activity programmes on the movement ability and social responsiveness of children with ASD and co-occurring learning disabilities. The study involved 17 students with ASD and learning disabilities participating in an adapted physical activity intervention over a 10-week period three times per week, in a special school setting. A non-active group (n = 7) with motor impairment and co-occurring learning disabilities was used as control. Quantitatively, movement ability was assessed using the MABC (Henderson and Sugden, 1992), and social responsiveness was assessed using the SRS (Constantino and Gruber, 2005). The intervention consisted of an obstacle course with a variety of fine, gross and organisational activities. Applied Behaviour Analysis (ABA) principles were used including 1:1 instruction, model and physical prompting, and reinforcement. Results indicated significant improvements occurred for the intervention group in ball skills, static and dynamic balance, social communication, social motivation and autistic mannerisms. In the qualitative analysis using the pupil evaluation checklist (Wright and Sugden, 1999) improvements occurred in physical, intellectual, social, emotional and attitude components for the intervention group. No changes occurred for the control group. Overall results indicated the benefits of ABA programmes in promoting movement ability and social responsiveness for children with ASD and co-occurring learning disabilities. Findings also indicated that appropriate support and training were essential for teachers and special needs assistants to deliver quality ABA programmes to this population and to children with other disabilities in an Irish context.

Todd and Reid (2006) investigated the outcomes of a physical activity intervention programme, using snowshoeing and walking/jogging for individuals with ASD. The programme was of 6 months' duration and included three teenagers diagnosed with ASD. A changing conditions design was used and included a self-monitoring board, verbal cuing and edible reinforcers. Results indicated that the distance walked/jogged/snowshoed increased, despite reductions in edible and verbal reinforcers. These results suggest that interventions can be successfully developed to promote sustained participation in physical activity for individuals with ASD.

In earlier studies Prupas and Reid (2001) examined the effects of exercise frequency on stereotypical behaviours in four children with developmental disabilities. The children ranged in age from 5–9 years. Two children displayed autistic characteristics and tendencies symptomatic of PDD-NOS, while the other two were diagnosed with ASD and Fragile X syndrome. A 6-week observation period where behaviours were confirmed and recorded occurred prior to the study. Two exercise frequencies of single and multiple daily walk/jog interventions were used. The multiple frequency condition was found to be the more effective intervention of the two, as the reduction in stereotypical behaviour was maintained throughout the day at different periods. Occasions where exercise was followed by only a modest change in stereotypical behaviours coincided with an unstructured environment, such as break time or free play. Observation in the classroom also suggested that, as the structure of the classroom increased, stereotypical behaviours decreased. The researchers stated that exercise, combined with a structured classroom, yielded an optimum decrease in stereotypical behaviours. Celeberti et al. (1997) examined the differential and temporal effects of antecedent exercise on the self-stimulatory behaviour of a 6-year-old child with ASD. The researchers examined the effects of walking versus jogging in suppressing self-stimulatory behaviour. The exercise programmes were carried out before classes of academic programmes and were of 6 minutes in duration. Self-stimulatory behaviours were separately tracked. The intervention period was of 3 weeks' duration. Findings indicated a decrease in physical self-stimulation and 'out-of-seat' behaviour after the jogging intervention only. A reduction in these behaviours occurred immediately after the jogging intervention and gradually increased, but did not return to baseline levels, over a 40-minute period. Positive effects have also been found with roller skating (Powers, Thibadeau and Rose, 1992), aerobic exercise (Bachman and Sluyter, 1988) and non-structured exercise (McGimsey and Favell, 1988). Schleien *et al.* (1987) investigated the effects of integrating children with ASD into a physical and recreational setting. The researchers sought to establish whether changes occurred in subjects' social, leisure and adaptive behaviour skills from pre- to post-physical activity programme treatment. Attitudes of typically developed peers towards children with disabilities were also assessed. Two children with severe ASD and 67 typically developed children participated in the study. The 3-week physical activity programme consisted of three 40-minute activity periods, including cooperative sports and games, swimming and gymnastics, followed by a 30-minute open recreation session. Children from the typically developed group volunteered to act as 'buddies' and were rotated on a weekly basis. Findings indicated positive increases occurred in appropriate play behaviour and positive orientation to play objects and peers. There were substantial decreases in inappropriate play behaviours. Attitudes towards the subjects with ASD from their typically developed peers revealed positive but insignificant improvement. Kern, Koegel and Dunlap (1984) examined the effects of mild versus vigorous exercise on stereotypical behaviours of three children with ASD.

The interventions used were jogging and ball skills, for 15-minute periods. A simultaneous-treatments design (Kazdin and Hartmann, 1978) was used, in which sessions of one condition (jogging) were alternated with sessions of the other (ball skills). The results showed that non-vigorous exercise had little effect on stereotypical behaviours, but vigorous exercise caused a decrease in stereotypical behaviours.

The effects of FMS interventions for this population is clearly verified in research. Further validated intervention studies addressing movement impairment issues are needed. Equally it is important to identify the effects of frequency, intensity and duration of such programmes. Interventions addressing issues of social impairment, for example, stereotypical behaviour, need to be conducted for longer periods and the effects of these interventions validated for maintenance and generalisation.

KEY POINTS

* Motor skill interventions are effective in addressing motor impairment for individuals with ASD.

* Benefits of increased frequency, intensity and duration effects are confirmed by research.

Comparative study of physical activity levels among children with and without ASD

This section includes:

* Physical activity levels of children with ASD

Physical activity research in children and youth with ASD is scarce and often contradictory (Wilczynski *et al.*, 2009). Current guidelines from the United States Department of Health and Human Services (USDHHS; Carlson *et al.*, 2010) recommend that children aged 6–17 years participate in a minimum of 60 minutes of moderate or vigorous physical activity (MVPA) every day. Although not the primary focus of their study, Ketcheson *et al.* (2016) found that both the control and experimental groups met or exceeded USDHHS recommendations for 60 minutes of MVPA per day. However, both groups spent the majority of their day (i.e. 8 hours) in sedentary activity. Tyler, MacDonald and Menear (2014) examined the physical activity and fitness of school-aged children with ASD in comparison to typically developing peers, and found significant between-group effects in strength, in sedentary, light, moderate and total MVPA. The researchers concluded that children with ASD were less physically active and fit than typically developing peers and that adapted physical activity programmes were one avenue with intervention potential to combat these lower levels of physical activity and fitness found in children with ASD. In a large cross-sectional study examining objective physical activity in youth with ASD, both the younger (aged 9–11 years) and the older (aged 12–18 years) groups met the current recommendations of 60 minutes of daily MVPA (MacDonald, Esposito and Ulrich, 2011). Further findings revealed an age-related decline in activity, where participants in the older group spent significantly more time per day in sedentary activity and significantly less time in MVPA. However, the findings of Bandini *et al.* (2013) measuring objective physical activity in young children with and without ASD (aged 3–11 years), indicated that 43 per cent of children with typical development met the minimum requirement of 60 minutes of daily MVPA compared to just 23 per cent of children with ASD. An earlier comparison study of physical activity levels between children with and without ASD by Sandt and Frey (2005) examined daily physical education, daily recess and after-school MVPA levels, between children with and without ASD. Findings indicated that there were no differences between children with and without ASD, at any physical activity setting. Both groups were more active during recess than after school. Children with ASD were similarly active in recess and physical education classes. The researchers indicated that many of the children with ASD acquired 60 minutes of physical activity overall per day, but this could potentially decrease with age, as opportunities for recess and physical education were eliminated.

KEY POINT

* Children with ASD are not as physically active as recommended.

Summary

Chapter 3 examined research on motor impairments, FMS interventions and physical activity levels of individuals with ASD. Difficulties with motor development were identified as early as infancy in individuals with ASD. Intervention studies were found to be effective in addressing motor impairment for this population. Physical activity levels of individuals with ASD were similar to those without the diagnosis, with both tending towards sedentary activities after school hours.

CHAPTER 4

Tools for Assessment of Fundamental Movement Skills of Individuals with ASD

Accurately assessing fundamental movement skills (FMS) of participants with autism spectrum disorder (ASD) can depend where on the spectrum the participant is. In relation to assessment tests, the movement assessment can be norm- or criterion-referenced. A norm-referenced test compares the child's performance to that of a normative group, and quantifies the child's movement skill competence. A criterion-referenced test compares the child's performance to predetermined criteria. A criterion-referenced test takes into account the qualitative aspects of the movements required to perform the movement skill item. A further form of movement skill assessment is through pupil monitoring instruments and is mainly used by teachers.

Many factors must be taken into account when deciding which method should be used for a particular assessment, including the aim of the assessment, characteristics of the participants and the resources available. There is an abundance of literature and studies dealing with the assessment of movement ability of adults and adolescents without disabilities, but unfortunately there is not a wealth of information when it comes to children, particularly children with a specific disability, such as ASD. Assessment tools that allow for a variety of measures, that is, quantitative (to establish definitive measures) and qualitative (to examine additional characteristics), must be considered so that clear and comprehensive findings can be established.

Explanation and justification of assessment tools available

To ensure comprehensive assessment in the identified area of movement ability, it is necessary to review assessment tools that deliver accurate findings for the population with ASD.

Assessment of movement ability of individuals with ASD

This section includes:

- Movement ability tests assist in screening, planning implementing and evaluating FMS programmes. However, not all tests are suitable for all children

- Specific tests of movement assessment include some of the following: Movement Assessment Battery for Children (MABC; Henderson, Sugden and Barnett, 2007a, 2007b; Henderson and Sugden, 1992), Peabody Developmental Motor Scales – Second Edition (PDMS-2; Folio and Fewell, 1983, 2000); Test of Gross Motor Development 2 (TGMD-2) (Ulrich, 1985), Bruininks–Osteretsky test (Bruininks, 1978) and the Manchester Motor Skills Assessment (MMSA; Bond *et al.*, 2007)

- Reflective Framework for Teaching and Learning in Physical Education (Tsangaridou and O'Sullivan, 1994)

MABC (Henderson and Sugden, 1992; updated Henderson *et al.*, 2007a, 2007b)

The Movement Assessment Battery for Children (MABC) is the common assessment tool of choice for children with movement difficulties in Ireland, the United Kingdom and throughout Europe (Henderson *et al.*, 2007a, 2007b). The original MABC by Henderson and Sugden (1992) has evolved from the popular Test of Motor Impairment by Stott, Moyes and Henderson (1984), later referred to as the TOMI – Henderson (Riggen, Ulrich and Ozmun, 1990), and was updated again in 2007. The MABC has 32 items organised by four age levels so that the general movement competence of a child can be assessed with eight items. These include manual dexterity (e.g. writing, cutting and peg boards), ball skills (e.g. catching and throwing at targets), static and dynamic balance (e.g. board balance, jumping and clapping and walking backwards) over a range of tasks. These tasks are carefully selected to be easy for most children in a designated age band. Performance in the test is recorded with raw scores converted into scaled scores, in order to ascertain where the child's performance lies, in relation to the standardisation sample. This can be done for individual items or for the total score (i.e. manual dexterity, ball skills and static and dynamic balance). A qualitative aspect of the test encourages the assessor to record how the child performs by using a series of descriptors (e.g. posture, ability to control hand movements). Both the test and MABC teacher checklist provide the guide to behavioural factors that may influence motor performance.

PDMS-2 (Folio and Fewell, 1983, 2000)

The Peabody Developmental Motor Scales, 2nd edn (PDMS-2) is a movement skill assessment tool that measures gross and fine movement skills. It focuses on assessment, intervention and treatment programming for children with disabilities. The test estimates a child's motor competence, the development of fine and gross motor movement skills, identifies deficits and evaluates progress. The PDMS-2 is a revision of the original and consists of six scales designed to assess movement skills of children from birth to six years of age. The gross movement subtests include reflexes, stationary performances, locomotion and object manipulation. The fine movement subtests include grasping and visual-motor integration. The total motor score is the sum of all six subtest scores. The PDMS-2 test has optimised reliability and validity with score criteria and illustrations included.

TGMD-2 (Ulrich, 1985, 2000)

The Test of Gross Motor Development, 2nd edn (TGDM-2) measures gross movement performance based on qualitative aspects of movement skills. The test can be used to identify delay in gross motor performance, for programme planning and to assess changes as a function of increasing age, experience, instruction or intervention. The TGDM-2 is a revision of the original Test of Gross Motor Development (TGMD), published in 1985 (Ulrich, 1985). The age range is 3–10 years. The test includes locomotion and object control skills with the sum of two performances representing the final score for each skill. The TGDM-2 also includes qualitative aspects in the assessment.

Currently, the TGMD-3 is finalising the normative data set so that norms may be published for general use. Publication of the TGMD-3 is expected soon (www.kines.umich.edu/tgmd3/).

BOTMP-BOT-2 (Bruininks, 1978; Bruininks and Bruininks, 2005)

The Bruininks-Oseretsky Test of Motor Proficiency (BOTMP) and its review the Bruininks-Oseretsky Test of Motor Proficiency, second edition (BOT-2) are tools to assess fine and gross movement skill development. They are used to identify individuals with mild to moderate motor coordination deficits. The test is suitable for individuals aged 4–21 years. The complete BOT-2 is divided into subtests including fine and gross motor skills, coordination and balance. A short form of the BOT-2 can be used as a screening tool to achieve rapid and easy scoring reflecting overall motor proficiency. The sum of scores results in a total motor composite. The test is recommended for motor impairment diagnosis, screening, placement decisions, development and evaluation of motor training programs and supporting research goals. The test is only obtainable by medical and paramedical professions.

MMSA (Bond *et al.*, 2007)

The MMSA is designed to be quick and easy for teaching staff and assistants to complete, with the dual purposes of informing group programme planning and demonstrating an individual child's progress following a period of intervention. Inter-rater reliability checks were conducted during initial assessments of 37 children in 11 schools. The MMSA comprised two appendices. Appendix 1 is designed for children aged between 4 and 6 years of age. Appendix 2 is designed for those aged 7–9 years old. Teachers mark students using a 4-point scale on each activity in fine, gross and organisational skill categories. The scoring system for the total was as follows: 0 = fail; a score of 1–10 = poor; 11–20 = fair; and finally 21–30 = good. Both teachers and special needs assistants report its ease of administration for both assessment and programme planning (Crawford *et al.*, 2012).

The Reflective Framework for Teaching and Learning in Physical Education (Tsangaridou and O'Sullivan, 1994)

The Reflective Framework for Teaching and Learning in Physical Education, designed by Tsangaridou and O'Sullivan (1994), provides a reflective tool with three approaches to promoting quality and in-depth reflection, including a reflective journal, video commentary and class observations. Each aspect of the framework has guiding questions to help the researcher/participant attain a deep and in-depth level of reflection, moving from descriptive to sensitising levels of reflection when assessing participation in FMS.

KEY POINTS

* All assessment tools are suitable to assess fine and gross motor skills of children on the spectrum.

* The Reflective Framework for Teaching and Learning in Physical Education provides a qualitative tool to consider FMS, using video, observation and journal entries with guiding questions for each.

Summary

This chapter explored specific tests of movement assessment as follows: the MABC (Henderson and Sugden, 1992; Henderson *et al.*, 2007a, 2007b); PDMS-2 (Folio and Fewell, 1983, 2000); TGMD-2 (Ulrich, 1985, 2000); BOTMP-BOT-2 (Bruininks, 1978; Bruininks and Bruininks, 2005); the MMSA (Bond *et al.*, 2007); and the Reflective Framework for Teaching and Learning in Physical Education (Tsangaridou and O'Sullivan, 1994). The tools used should be based on understanding the individual, the task and the environment.

CHAPTER 5

Promoting and Maintaining Participation in FMS Programmes for Individuals with ASD

This chapter examines how to establish and maintain effective participation in fundamental movement skills (FMS)-based programmes for children and adults on the spectrum (Crawford *et al.*, 2013; Reid and Collier, 2002; Reid and O'Connor, 2003; Reid, O'Connor and Lloyd, 2003).

Assessment for FMS selection for individuals with autism spectrum disorder (ASD)

This section includes:

- Understanding the individual

- Understanding the environment

- Understanding the task

Research on FMS programme planning for individuals on the spectrum indicates that ecological interventions are the most effective, where adaptations to the teaching and learning approach and to the environment are used to facilitate learning

(Block, 2000; Chambers and Sugden, 2006; Crawford *et al.*, 2013; Henderson and Sugden, 2007; Reid and O'Connor, 2003). According to Reid and O'Connor (2003):

> Content for instruction should be based on the interests, needs and supports of the individual, rather than a label of ASD. The goal is not therapy but enhancing the ability and desire to engage in independently selected physical activity. (Reid and O'Connor, 2003, p.20)

Block (2000) recommends an ecological or 'top-down' approach in relation to FMS selection. This approach takes account of the individual's interests, abilities and probability of repeated exposure to the activity, in the current and future life of the individual. It also involves an examination of what is currently available in the individual's school, home and community setting (Kozub, 2001). Reid and O'Connor (2003) indicate the following specifics that need addressing in relation to FMS and physical activity selection and, over time, these key tenets of activity selection have not changed:

- Choice accommodates individual interests and strengths.

- Activities are age appropriate.

- Peer interest in community and culture: establishing what peer interests are in the community.

- Parent interest, so that compliance in activities is at a maximum.

- Social and cognitive demands of FMS should reflect the comprehension and tolerance of each individual with ASD.

- Consideration of competition and cooperation, where cooperative FMS-based activities may be appropriate.

- Assessment for FMS and physical activity programme planning should be viewed as part of a continuous process where the interrelated nature of the individual, tasks and the environment needs to be considered.

Understanding the individual

Understanding the individual with ASD is a key component of the assessment process, and involves liaison with parents and professionals, who play an integral role in the individual's life. Reinforcers, motivators and potentially stressful environments can all be identified (Reid and O'Connor, 2003). Individual areas of strength are important. Combined with family interests, individual strengths can provide positive and successful starting points, which increase the likelihood of the individual with ASD remaining with the FMS-based activity (Kozub, 2001; Simpson and Zionts, 1999). Where possible, the assessor should communicate directly with the individual, using the preferred modality of communication, for example, iPad, Picture Exchange Communication System (PECS) folder, visual aids, communication board, etc. (Crawford *et al.*, 2013).

Understanding the environment

Understanding the environment is essential so that potential interferences can be identified. It is important to establish if the individual is hypo- or hypersensitive to sounds, smells, tastes, lighting or large numbers of people present (Simpson and Zionts, 1999). Identifying, minimising and, if possible, eliminating environmental issues is a key component to promoting participation for the individual with ASD (Grandin, 1996; Wing, 2002).

Understanding the task

The individual's understanding of the task is also a key element of the assessment process. It is essential that the assessment consider the individual's learning style (Staples *et al.*, 2011). A task analysis of the target skill is also essential, so that each component part of that skill is also assessed (Block, 2000). Assessment should also consider the individual's reaction and interaction with others, and any unusual behaviour should be noted (Reid and O'Connor, 2003). Finally, the assessment process should identify current and future recreation activities, environments and specific skills required for participation in activities. New skills should be the focus of learning experiences, while acquired skills should be part of a maintenance programme (Block, 2000; Reid and O'Connor, 2003).

KEY POINTS

* Understanding the individual: consider each person, family, community and support holistically.

* Understanding the environment: consider sensitivity to sensory stimuli.

* Understanding the task: know the individual's learning style and the components of the task involved.

Intervention and programme planning for individuals with ASD

As stated earlier, due to the heterogeneity of individuals with ASD, individualised approaches are essential when designing an FMS intervention (Jordan, Jones and Murray, 1998; Reid and O'Connor, 2003; Wing, 2002). From consideration of the characteristics of ASD and subsequent interventions available, some definite pointers arise in intervention delivery for facilitators.

This section includes these key indicators from Reid and O'Connor (2003) and, more recently, Crawford *et al.* (2013) as follows:

- Individual instruction

- Low student to teacher ratio

- Task variation

- Stimulus generalisation of learning

- Self-determination

- Structured learning environment

- Physical structure: schedules, work systems, and routines and transitions

Individual instruction

Individual instruction considers the likes and dislikes of the individual so that FMS-based activities are enjoyable, meaningful and likely to lead to success (Wing, 2002). Particular preferences are considered and accommodated, for example, if a child has a preference for a specific ball and bat it may help sustain interest in the activity.

Low student to teacher/facilitator ratio

Low student to teacher/facilitator ratio and one-to-one interactions are often beneficial, especially for individuals with co-occurring learning disabilities or behaviour issues especially when beginning an FMS programme (Crawford *et al.*, 2013). Using the 'buddy system' to promote peer interaction and to provide demonstrations and guidance can be effective (Jordan *et al.*, 1998). Peers can demonstrate activities (catching, throwing, jumping), assist with physical (help shoot for a basket) and verbal prompts (throw ball), and act as a partner. The special needs assistant (SNA) has been found to have a major role in promoting participation for the individual with ASD in an educational setting, giving support, reinforcing instruction and prompting as necessary (Crawford *et al.*, 2013; Department of Education and Science, 2001; Ring, 2006).

Task variation

An alternative approach to constant task instruction for the individual with ASD is that of task variation. Task variation involves teaching new skills, interspersed with skills already mastered, for example, catching a ball is followed by kicking to a target (Crawford *et al.*, 2013; Henderson and Sugden, 2007; Weber and Thorpe, 1992). This approach is associated with decreased aggression and self-stimulation (Dunlap, 1984). It has also been found to be appropriate for younger children with ASD and those with co-occurring learning disabilities where attention and concentration is often difficult (O'Connor, French and Henderson, 2000). O'Connor *et al.* (2000) also recommended that practice trials of new skills could be interspersed with previously mastered skills, every 2–3 minutes.

Stimulus generalisation of learning

Stimulus generalisation of learning has been identified as requiring different cues, materials, people and settings (Heflin and Alberto, 2001). FMS-based activities of interest to the individual with ASD and especially those that are also of family interest should be included to promote generalisation to a variety of settings (Crawford *et al.*, 2013; Kozub, 2001). Using a variety of balls, targets and shapes helps promote generalisation and reduce fixations on any one dimension of equipment and indeed the environment (Schultheis, Boswell and Decker, 2000).

Self-determination

Self-determination, where the individual with ASD makes choices, is an essential component of intervention delivery (Crawford *et al.*, 2013; Reid and O'Connor, 2003). Individuals who chose their own activities, locations and materials were more likely to engage in those activities and have less behaviour issues according to Newman *et al.* (2002). Self-management and personal goal setting are other aspects of self-determination. The individual with ASD is encouraged to count laps, jumps on the trampoline, etc., and is assisted to record the same so that new targets can be set (Todd and Reid, 2006).

Structured learning environment

A structured learning environment is identified as a necessary component of intervention delivery for individuals with ASD (Crawford *et al.*, 2013; Mesibov, Browder and Kirkland, 2002; O'Connor *et al.*, 2000; Reid and O'Connor, 2003). These researchers indicate that structure provides clarity and predictability to learning, assists in transitions, helps individuals to reorganise and fosters independence. Structure is also advocated as reducing and eliminating difficult behaviours (Mesibov and Shea, 2003).

Physical structure

Physical structure involves reducing distractions and increasing time on task, as much as possible. Schultheis *et al.* (2000) stated that room dividers, covered windows and 'wait' chairs/mats for programme participants were effective in promoting independent behaviour, increased time on task and fostering emotional security.

Schedules

The use of schedules showing a sequence of activities is also advocated to provide structure and guidance, promote independence, reduce attention difficulties, be used as a communication aid to indicate what comes next and make transitioning from one skill to another easy (Crawford *et al.*, 2013; Mesibov *et al.*, 2002; Schopler and Mesibov, 2000; Schultheis *et al.*, 2000).

Work systems

Work systems provide precise instructions to guide the individual with ASD and are often in picture form. Each task is broken down into component parts and each component forms part of the work system (Reid and O'Connor, 2003). For example, FMS ball skills would have visuals of each skill to be practised, a visual of the hall, work stations and a visual of the stretch programme for before and after.

Routines and transitions

Routines and transitions are essential components of FMS intervention planning and delivery. These help to increase familiarity and reduce anxiety for the individual with ASD (Crawford *et al.*, 2013; Jordan *et al.*, 1998). Reid and O'Connor (2003) recommend that physical activity facilitators start and finish lessons in a consistent manner, for example, warm up and cool down sessions. Myles (2001) and Crawford *et al.* (2013) suggest that 'priming', where an activity is introduced prior to its use, might be useful when the individual is making the transition from one task to another. This can be done using the iPad/Mobile Digital Technology (MDT) approach.

KEY POINTS

- Individual instruction: consider likes, dislikes and preferences.

- Low student to teacher ratio: 1:1 and increase as tolerated.

- Task variation: teach new skills and intersperse with those already mastered.

- Stimulus generalisation of learning: as skills are mastered generalise to different environments.

- Self-determination: ensure choice to maintain motivation.

- Structured learning environment: provides predictability, use visuals as necessary.

- Physical structure (schedules, work systems and routines and transitions): reduce distractions, provide visual support, establish a routine and prepare for transitions.

The ASD/FMS support kit

To ensure the delivery of FMS sessions runs as smoothly as possible, it is important to make contingency plans in terms of having additional support equipment and, ideally, personnel available. A support kit can contain a variety of equipment that can be used to help with self-regulation, proprioception and managing anxiety as the needs arise. It could include:

- Time out mat: have this set up in a quiet area of the hall for any student to take time out or a breather as necessary.

- A set of light weights: these can be used under supervision for arm curls to aid regulation as necessary.

- TheraBand: this can be used for proprioceptive stretching and to provide proprioceptive feedback as required.

- An iPad/android/laptop/mobile digital appliance: an opportunity to review the skill can be used to provide visual prompts, reduce anxiety and as a communication aid before, during or after FMS sessions.

- A ball: one-to-one bouncing, throwing and catching can be interspersed as a regulatory break that provides proprioceptive feedback in a programme.

- A skipping rope: this can be used for skipping activities or as a tether to support the running of laps for regulation.

- A selection of activity cards: these can be used as teaching and learning tools, communication aids and visual prompts, or to reinforce skill acquisition.

- Pens/pencils/paint set: these can be used for some fine motor work to end a session, revisit what happened in the session, include some incidental teaching and learning regarding colours, shapes, sizes and FMS activities, and to get feedback from the participant about the session.

KEY POINT

* The ASD/FMS support kit should contain general and person-centred equipment to establish regulation and proprioception and reduce anxiety.

Maximising FMS acquisition

Researchers indicate that maximising skill acquisition and promoting participation is reliant on the following factors (Block, 2000; Crawford *et al.*, 2013; Mesibov *et al.*, 2002; Reid and O'Connor, 2003; Schopler and Mesibov, 2000; Schultheis *et al.*, 2000):

- Allowing time for familiarity.

- Promoting eye contact.

- Use of clear language.

- Being aware of sensory preferences and overselectivity.

- Balancing social skills training and physical activity objectives.

- The use of Applied Behaviour Analysis (ABA).

- Use of recording format.

- Use of prompts.

- The use of reinforcements.

- Use of incidental teaching.

- Use of Pivotal Response Training (PRT).

- Use of Treatment and Education of Autistic and related Communication Handicapped Children (TEACCH) components.

- Use of MDT/video analysis.

- Use of proprioceptive stretches pre- and post-FMS programme.

Allowing time for familiarity

Take the child to the venue/hall/outdoor facility for the FMS-based physical activity session several times prior to actually starting the session. Allow the child to walk around the venue, so that they may become familiar with the area prior to starting the activity. They may wish to touch the wall perimeter, examine the layout of the area. Be aware that they may need to become familiar with sounds that may echo, birds/animals in the outdoors, other people using the facility or smells associated with a new facility. They should be introduced to the toilet facilities and how to be safe in a public facility. Chat about the new premises/facilities with enthusiasm at home. With permission, video the area so that they can revise/revisit it in their own time. Staff members should be introduced one by one. Allow the child to initiate contact when ready. If others are assisting you with your FMS programme ensure they are familiar with the child's likes, dislikes, issues that may arise and safety issues.

> **Case scenario: coach of an 11-year-old boy with moderate ASD and learning disabilities**
> Michael was joining our football training programme. Beforehand we had asked his mum to complete the individualised personal profile so we could transition him as easily as possible to the group. They visited the field and dressing room on several occasions before actually participating. Videos of the sessions in action were taken as were photos of us and the surrounds. Mum could then use these to prepare him to come along with his gear. We also gave him a football to bring home and practise kicking and throwing. He was very happy to finally come and join the team.

Promoting eye contact

Introduce the child to other buddies, participants, family members and facilitators participating in the programme as appropriate. Encourage the child to look at each individual prior to activity. Be at eye level with the child and encourage others to do likewise when communicating initially. Promote choice of activity and respond to the child's choice. This will provide more potential for positive eye contact and engagement. Allow the child space: do not try and force eye contact; they may need time to assimilate to new people, tasks and surroundings. Praise and reinforce positive eye contact, for example, 'good looking'. Use minimal words/short sentences to reduce anxiety around information processing and allow the participant to engage visually.

> **Case scenario: teacher of a 5-year-old boy with moderate ASD**
> I worked at limiting too much sensory overload for John so he could concentrate on looking and tracking others visually. Sometimes he would ask to use ear plugs to make this easier. When speaking, I would move in front of him. I insisted all our students and teachers did likewise. I also encouraged people to get down to his level when they spoke to him and to keep words to a minimum initially. It became automatic with us all. Now, sometimes if he is tired, the eye contact is not as consistent.

Use of clear language

Use the appropriate communication modality for the child, that is, visual aids such as PECS, iPad, visual schedules. Ensure these are brought to all activity sessions. Ensure coaches/teachers/tutors are familiar with the aids. Use two- or three-word sentences during activities, depending on the child's comprehension, and increase the word count accordingly. Gain the child's attention first by calling their name before activities. Do not give complicated or long instructions during activities/games time. Go through the skill breakdown in clear language, until the child understands what is expected of them. Build on comprehension at the child's pace. Use the video demonstrations on www.getautismactive.com both at home and at the session to reinforce what is involved. It is also useful to video the participant doing the FMS so they can revisit them at home/school for practice and refinement purposes.

Case scenario: mother of a 16-year-old boy with moderate ASD, moderate learning disabilities and severe speech and language disorder

We started out with PECS but quickly moved to the iPad and began building up banks of video demos for all activities as we went. It worked really well. Tommy would automatically take out the iPad to remind himself what he had covered and how to do it again. It's a great measuring tool of improvement and success now as we tick accomplishing each of the skills one by one.

Being aware of sensory preferences and overselectivity

Complete a sensory profile on the participant with parents/ carers and the occupational therapist to identify what sensory preferences or issues they may have. The sensory profile needs to be updated regularly. Some participants with ASD may be hypo- or hypersensitive to particular stimuli and it is important to identify these before starting a session to limit issues around difficulties that may occur. These sensory preferences may change over time, and a participant who initially presented as hyposensitive to sound may become hypersensitive to that particular sound and become disruptive when it is used.

Case scenario: parent of a 9-year-old girl with mild ASD

Mary really disliked having her head touched. We were called to the unit (ASD unit in mainstream school) as she had lost it in the yard when one of her 'buddies' touched her head playing tag. We hadn't stressed it enough at the previous meeting, I suppose. The other children got an awful fright too. We worked with the OT (occupational therapist) on brushing and deep pressure programmes to help her overcome it.

Balancing social skills training and physical activity objectives

Where addressing FMS development is an important goal, social skills training can also take place. Start with one-to-one interaction and slowly increase to small groups as tolerated. Encourage the participant to respond when addressed. Introduce the participant with ASD to each of the other participants and encourage acknowledging others. Encourage turn taking in activities, 'wait your turn'. Reward good waiting and good turn taking. Encourage the child to assist with setting up of the FMS circuit/activities with others and to tidy up afterwards. This will go from parallel engagement where the participant will concentrate on the chore to actually becoming aware of and engaging with buddies and team mates, who can be encouraged to initiate engagement. After a session try and include a snack/drink at the end for all to ensure the social aspect of engagement is maximised. Encourage the participant to draw a picture/write a story of the activity. Build a book of buddies and events that they can return to.

Case scenario: mother of a 17-year-old boy with moderate ASD, moderate learning disability and severe speech and language disorder

Tomás was always a runner: at the start, up at night running up and down the hall, you name it. I decided to turn it to our advantage and began to take him out for short walks and run home. The distance increased and he really seemed to like it. After a few months of just the two of us, I asked my friends if they would join us on Sunday mornings and they agreed. We soon had a routine of long Sunday runs, followed by breakfast together. In time Tomás was setting the table for the others. Funnily, when he ran his first half-marathon with the group, one of the gang was struggling at the end to keep up. He told us to head on without him but Tomás refused to leave him, insisting we all stay together and finish together. What about that for loyalty born from running?

Use of ABA

As outlined earlier ABA is commonly used as a teaching methodology/technique with children and adults on the spectrum. Break skills down into smaller parts as necessary, for example: extending the child's arm to catch a ball; throwing a ball as far as possible until success is achieved; consistent use of a ball and introducing variety as FMS development is progressing. Work one to one with the child until they achieve fluency, that is, can participate in the skill/activity without prompting. Reward/reinforce each success with a treat and/ or praise. Use repetition until a skill is mastered. Ensure the environment is uncluttered when teaching new activities, keeping distractions to a minimum. Provide demonstrations and prompts as necessary.

Case scenario: father of an 18-year-old boy with mild ASD and mild learning disabilities

We were using ABA from when Aidan was 3 or 4 years old. We learned the basics through workshop training organised by an amazing dad of a young boy with ASD. So whenever we wanted to teach Aidan a new skill, we would look up Catherine Maurice's book *Let Me Hear Your Voice* and use it as our guide. We bought a timer and counted how often he did each skill or part of a skill in a minute and graphed our findings. Aidan learned to catch, throw, jump and run by breaking each of the skills down, with us working one to one with him and using constant repetition and reinforcement. We still use ABA 15 years later and it still works. You get used to breaking everything down and finally putting it all back together again.

Use of recording format

Begin by recording what the child can do, for example, catch, throw, run and jump. Quantify how much of each skill your child can do, for example, ten throws to a hoop, ten laps of the track. Are they using arms, trunk or legs with different activities? Document short-term goals and build towards long-term goals. Keep a daily/weekly diary of activities participated in: note details of your child, the activity and the environment. Record the child's reaction to and engagement with others. Use a written diary, voice recorder, video with iTouch, iPad, video recorder, pictures. Encourage the child to write up/draw/ record their experiences also, these can be used to reinforce positive activities and promote recurrence. Keep a record of reinforcers and note if primary reinforcers (i.e. food, objects) are being replaced by secondary reinforcers (i.e. praise). Record if the child has difficulties or appears unhappy with any particular activity. Note what happened before the activity, during the activity and after the activity.

Case scenario: mother of a 7-year-old girl with mild ASD

As a family we always videoed our kids playing outdoors, you know, the usual. When Anne was diagnosed with ASD, we were able to look back and see the delays that were there, especially in her walking and climbing the stairs. When we were encouraged to promote FMS programmes we were told by the facilitator to video all activities and use them to set new targets. It was great advice, now we use the iPhone all the time. Its non-invasive, can pick up spontaneous activities, engagement and different successes. Anne likes looking at them too. Parents of children with ASD should be encouraged to record how their children are doing in different settings; how they interact with others and if they do well.

Use of prompts

A prompt is used to elicit a response but should be faded when not needed. Verbal prompts can be used depending on the child's comprehension of language. Record prompts to help the child understand what comes next. Use visual prompts where possible, for example, pictures, schedules, video and the written word. Physical prompts can be used to give the child the 'feel' for an activity, for example, extending the child's arm to catch a ball. Model prompting involves demonstrating an activity firstly in its entirety and then breaking it down and modelling in parts until the child correctly responds to each part. Reinforce success but prepare to fade prompts as the child participates more.

Case scenario: swim teacher of a 14-year-old boy with severe ASD and learning disabilities

I was working on teaching John how to swim. I used a visual schedule showing him what the day involved. I then had a work schedule to break down the actual skill of swimming from arriving at the pool to getting him into the water. I model prompted each part of the swim as my swim tutor had taught me. I used to move John's arm through each of the skills, getting him used to the feel of it both in the water and out of it. The more he practised the fewer prompts he needed both verbally and physically. To me prompting is essential for the child's success and it's never too late to use them.

Use of reinforcers

Reinforcers can be important tools to promote the child to engage in FMS-based physical activities, so choose wisely. Ask the child! Consider the child's age, interests, likes and dislikes. Reinforcers can be primary/tangible (i.e. material objects), or secondary (i.e. activity-based or social-based). Always accompany reinforcers with praise. Know what reinforcers you will use before embarking on activities. Reinforcers should only be used if the target activity has been completed. At the beginning reinforcers should be immediate, with delays between activity and reinforcement being introduced as tolerated.

Case scenario: mother of a 17-year-old boy with moderate ASD, moderate learning disability and severe speech and language disorder

Over the years I've seen Tomás's reinforcers change from his favourite sweets, when he was very young, to going for a swim now he is older. I used to cut jelly tots into tiny pieces and, whenever he achieved success at a task, I'd reward him. Each time he got a sweet, I'd praise him, being specific as to what he had succeeded at, for example, good throwing. He loved praise and would smile at any enthusiastic encouragement. Soon we were able to replace some of the jelly tots with praise. I also introduced a star board and encouraged Tomás to earn a star with each additional lap or jump he achieved. He loved this and it also helped his counting. His most recent reinforcer is his love of having a shower. He now looks to go running each day and on the way back he talks about his shower. I use it as a positive, healthy reinforcer. Parents should monitor what motivates their children and build on skill development with their individualised reinforcers. Make a list; watch what makes them light up. All children like tangible or edible reinforcers at the start but they will learn to work for praise, especially as they get older.

Use of incidental teaching

Learning in other areas can be incorporated into any physical activity programme. Encourage the child to monitor their own progress, for example, counting laps, successful catches, throws, jumps. Use the changing environment to comment on other aspects of daily life, for example, weather, animals/birds outdoors. Avail yourself of opportunities to promote use of vocabulary, sentences and develop comprehension. Develop opportunities to engage in activities with others promoting social interaction. Concepts of size, shape, rules can all be explored through activity. Body awareness can be developed: labelling body parts, changing direction, feeling the impact of activity on bones, joints and posture.

Case scenario: father of a 12 year old boy with moderate ASD

We live by the ocean and I take Cathal walking there several days a week. While we're walking I choose different routes across rocks, grass and sand. This really helps his posture, coordination and balance. We chat about the weather, the number of people on the beach, comment on the different activities going on, for example, surfing, sailing and swimming. We talk about the Atlantic Ocean and the countries it touches. I am constantly teaching and Cathal is constantly learning while engaging in activity; it's our endless blackboard! Activity provides all round opportunity for incidental teaching.

Use of PRT

Pivotal Response Training (PRT) is a useful tool to consider when engaging in activity. PRT considers those activities that will motivate the child to engage, for example, they enjoy water so will run so they can have a bath/shower. PRT looks at activities that promote the child to respond to multiple cues, for example, running outside promotes use of seeing, hearing, smell and instruction. PRT aims to promote the child's social interaction, for example, catching and throwing games with a buddy. PRT seeks to promote self-regulation for the child, for example, enhanced feeling of wellbeing and 'happy in their own skin' after a game of football.

Case scenario: brother of a 13-year-old boy with mild ASD

I enrolled John in the Special Olympics athletics team. I wanted him to be a part of something that would involve activity and training. I also wanted to give him the chance to meet others. It has been incredible what we have all gotten from this. John is motivated to train, has friends, can tolerate crowds, noise, and is much calmer and more regulated after training sessions. He and all of us have also had the experience of succeeding and winning gold.

Use of TEACCH components

TEACCH uses a highly structured environment: distractions are reduced. The physical environment is actively organised, for example, an obstacle course is clearly set up with each area of equipment clearly marked. Skills are broken down into small parts; for example, start with dipping toes in the pool until child is comfortable to submerge with assistance. Visual schedules indicate what the activity session involves, for example, 'Drive to park, kick football, have picnic, return home'. Work schedules further break this down, for example, 'Take ball from car, place on the ground, swing with right foot, kick ball and score a goal'. Routine is integral to the success of the programme; that is, be consistent when planning and delivering a programme.

Case scenario: mother of an 8-year-old girl with moderate ASD and learning disabilities

We have been using TEACCH for the past 3 years with Mona. First we have our daily visual schedule that's like a timetable. Activity of some kind is a part of every day and Mona chooses which activity she wants for each day and we put the icon on the board. Once the activity is completed she takes the icon off the board. We use the work schedule to break down any new activity. This summer Mona joined a surf camp for children with ASD. We did a work schedule of pictures, starting with the beach, the surf board, the wetsuit, surfers, carrying the board to the water, lying on the board with support and coming in from the water. We also used the iPhone to video Mona on the board and she can look back at it after each session. We did warm up sessions beforehand, jogging up and down the beach and then doing the stretches. We finished off with a similar cool down and kept the routine consistent. The structure and routine of TEACCH really suits Mona. The whole family is used to it.

Use of MDT/video analysis

The use of any MDT device provides the opportunity to record baseline skills and progression over time, and provides a communication tool to help with reinforcement and feedback. The recording of short video clips also provides a tool for motivation to practise and improve on FMS development both for the participant and family. Video clips can also be used for incidental teaching and learning opportunities, as the movements, the environment, the equipment and other participants can also be talked about together after the sessions. It can also provide the participant and family with an incentive to keep going when progress learning a new skill is slow.

> **Case scenario: parent of a 20-year-old man with ASD in a day service setting**
> I was delighted when they started recording the sessions. I could see what was happening and we could practise the same programme at home. Michael loved taking out the videos to look at himself and label different things going on. We then progressed to typing and writing what he was seeing, which was an added bonus. We can look back now and see how far he has come.

Use of proprioceptive stretches pre- and post-FMS programme

The use of proprioceptive stretches provides the individual with ASD with appropriate feedback to proprioceptors of the body. This further contributes to an overall feeling of regulation and reduces tension throughout the body. Following a structured stretching routine is essential both pre- and post-FMS delivery. A sample proprioceptive stretching programme can be found on www.getautismactive.com.

Again the programme comes with a visual demonstration and voiceover prompt for each stretch.

Case scenario: special needs assistant supporting a 12-year-old boy with ASD in a mainstream setting

I really wanted to encourage Alan to participate in physical activities as he was putting on weight. Mum wasn't too bothered either way. I did the getautismactive workshop and learned the stretches properly. We then began to use them every day in class before and after the FMS programme. They worked wonders in term of keeping him engaged and he seemed to need the support to stretch, whether it was the need for feedback or the clear demonstrations. I think it made all the difference in keeping him in the programme.

KEY POINTS

* Allowing time for familiarity: visit the venue several times, meet staff members and get accustomed to the environment.

* Promoting eye contact: be at child's level, reduce anxiety and use communication modality.

* Use of clear language: short sentences and personalised communication aid.

* Being aware of sensory preferences and overselectivity: establish hypo- and hypersensitivities to sensory stimuli.

* Balancing social skills training and physical activity objectives: ensure there is opportunity to socialise with others.

* The use of Applied Behaviour Analysis: break skills down, use reinforcers.

* Use of recording formats: chart progress – can be written, video or other.

* Use of prompts: use verbal, visual or physical prompts as necessary.

* The use of reinforcements: use individualised reinforcers, moving from tangible to secondary as progressing.

* Use of incidental teaching: use opportunity to teach new topics.

* Use of PRT: teach new skills simultaneously.

* Use of TEACCH components: use structure and visuals.

* Use of MDT/video analysis: use video, audio, mobile devices.

* Use of proprioceptive stretches pre- and post-FMS programme: provide proprioceptive feedback.

Summary

Chapter 5 explored promoting and maintaining participation in physical activity for children with ASD. It identified the need for detailed assessment for activity selection. An ecological approach to physical activity participation for individuals with ASD was recommended, which considered the interrelated nature of the individual, the task and the environment. Intervention programmes and planning need to address individual instruction, low student to teacher ratio, task variation, stimulus generalisation of learning, self-determination, structured learning environment and, finally, routines and transitions. Research on specific instructional methods allowed time for familiarity, promoted eye contact, used clear language, accommodated sensory preferences and over selectivity, balanced social skills training and physical activity objectives, used ABA, promoted incidental teaching, accommodated PRT, used TEACCH components and principles, adapted tasks and built success experiences and ensured the individual with ASD was motivated to participate. In relation to findings on activity selection, programme intervention and planning, many areas need to be addressed; these involve time, extra support staff and additional training of professionals involved, so that optimum participation occurs for individuals with ASD.

CHAPTER 6

www.getautismactive.com
Bringing it all together

Getautismactive is an online programme designed to enhance the quality of life for children and adults with autism spectrum disorder (ASD) by providing a training programme to develop and deliver the alphabet of movement. A number of fundamental movement skills (FMS) were chosen for the programme to include balance, ball bouncing, ball rolling, catching, dodging, forward roll, hitting a ball with a bat, hopping, horizontal jump, jumping from a height, kicking, leaping, overarm throw, running, skipping, sliding, static balance, vertical jump and volleying.

The basis of the programme is that if individuals with ASD learn and refine the FMS outlined, they will have increased self-efficacy, and feel more competent and confident to participate in quality physical activity, and thus avail themselves of the many benefits this participation affords. This includes the opportunity to be physically healthy, to socialise with others, to feel emotionally connected and to enjoy an endorphin release. Moreover, the risks associated with sedentary lifestyles will be reduced – obesity, hypertension and depression to mention but a few.

The programme embraces the principles and practices outlined in the previous chapters. These include taking an eclectic approach to teaching and learning skills for individuals on the spectrum, using a variety of teaching and learning methodologies and tools, and also taking opportunities for incidental teaching and learning. The principles include Applied Behaviour Analysis (ABA), Treatment and Education of Autistic and related Communication Handicapped Children (TEACCH), Pivotal Response Training (PRT), use of video, use of Mobile Digital Technology (MDT) and key aspects of reflective practice.

The programme is structured as follows:

- Each movement skill is broken down into component parts in the identifying features section.

- A video demonstration is provided for each skill.

- Voiceover prompts for the key teaching and learning points are included.

- Sample incidental teaching and learning points are included for each skill chosen.

- Proprioceptive stretches are included for pre- and post-sessions.

The format for programme delivery is as follows:

- Ensure the ASD/FMS support kit is available.

- Start off with a warm up and include the stretches in the stretches section.

- Watch the video of the skill.

- Demonstrate the skill.

- Ask the participant to imitate the skill.

- Video the participant doing the skill.

- Ask the participant to repeat each skill five times.

- Include at least three skills to be learnt and one from each category, for example, locomotor, manipulation and balance.

- Skills that are similar can be taught together, for example, catching and throwing.

- Use block practice of each skill to begin with and then extend to random practice in a game situation.

- Start off with 1:1 engagement initially until the rudiments of each skill are developed and then extend to include others as tolerated.

- Use the recorded video after training as a tool to further refine the skill and to provide the opportunity for further teaching and learning in relation to commenting on the skill, who, when, how and where it happened.

- Include and develop opportunities to challenge the development of new skills and the refinement of those already learnt.

- The more often a skill is practised, the more intensive the practice and the longer the practice, the greater the chance of success.

- Ask family to provide opportunities to engage in the skills in home, community and sports settings.

- Building a bank of video clips provides the participant, family, teachers and practitioners with a record of progress of skill development over time and may motivate a whole-family approach to participation.

The online programme includes a printable handbook, a sample of which follows. This affords the opportunity to record progress and list any relevant comments for each session. The reflective framework provides a guide to consider what worked well, what needed to be adjusted or amended and what to include in the next session.

Sample from workbook: catching: identifying features

	Sessions						
	1	2	3	4	5	6	7
No avoidance reaction							
Eyes follow ball into hands							
Arms are held relaxed at sides, and forearms are held in front of body							
Arms give on contact to absorb force of the ball							
Arms adjust to flight of ball							
Thumbs are held in opposition to each other							
Hands grasp ball in a well-timed, simultaneous motion							
Fingers grasp more effectively							

Additional learning opportunities

	Sessions						
	1	2	3	4	5	6	7
What is the girl doing?							
Show me catching high							
Show me catching low							
What is the girl moving?							
What colour is the ball?							
What shape is the ball?							

Comments:

_____

_____

_____

_____

_____

_____

_____

_____

_____

Sample reflective journal

1. Describe in detail one significant event that happened during your session or describe the session itself. It may be significant because it was something that excited you, bothered you, made you rethink your intentions/beliefs or made you realise that your intentions/beliefs were sound.

2. Analysis of the session and the programme.

   a. Specify why this event/session was significant.

   b. Explain how and why you reacted to this event/session.

   c. What did you learn from this event/session?

   d. How do you plan to follow up regarding this event/session?

The website also includes a blog of updated events, success stories and research findings. An online course to train as a getautismactive coach is proposed for the near future (2018).

Additional ASD/physical activity-related books are available to download from the books section and will be updated on an ongoing basis. The www.getautismaware.com website is currently being developed to promote autism awareness in family, community and business settings.

Summary

The getautismactive online programme (www.getautismactive. com) provides a clear guide to developing FMS for children and adults on the spectrum. The programme incorporates best practice in relation to developing movement skills for this population while embracing validated teaching and learning methodologies throughout.

Conclusions and Future Directions Identified

Conclusions and overall recommendations for future research, policy and practice in the areas of autism spectrum disorder (ASD) and fundamental movement skills (FMS) are now considered.

Research in the field of ASD and FMS needs to be promoted and developed both at national and international levels. This should include intervention studies addressing timing, duration, frequency and intensity of programmes for individuals on the spectrum. Research needs to consider the impact of age, the influence of co-occurring learning disabilities and indeed other co-occurring morbidities. The factors that influence the participation rates of individuals with ASD in physical activity also need to be empirically investigated.

Current research in the field of ASD tends to be oriented towards those on the less severe end of the spectrum. Those on the more severe end of the spectrum and with co-occurring learning disabilities need to be researched too, especially given the prevalence of both occurring together.

As regards programme facilitation, issues of lack of knowledge and lack of experience working with participants on the spectrum need to be addressed at undergraduate/pre-service level at third level institutes. Equally, teachers and other professionals currently working in the area of FMS programme planning and delivery need to be provided with appropriate in-service and practical workshops to support theoretical materials. Quality university-validated courses should be made available to those who wish to undertake more detailed study in this particular area. The training of special needs assistants/ classroom assistants (SNAs) is also an area that warrants attention.

Appropriate supportive educational materials need to be developed and readily available – similar to the getautismactive online initiative. These could include online content, DVDs, visual aids and modified/adapted equipment in a variety of shapes and sizes.

Whole-school/whole-practice/whole-community approaches need to be fostered and developed. This ensures issues of inclusion and delivery of quality programmes embrace both a top-down and a bottom-up approach and ripple throughout the school/therapeutic and general community settings. Both individuals with ASD and their typically developed peers hence learn and develop the tenets of quality movement, fair play and equality for all together. The forthcoming www.getautismaware.com programme will seek to address this ethos in both individual and collective settings.

Existing interventions and methodologies for those with ASD need to be empirically validated, so that parents and professionals can make informed choices as to what interventions are appropriate for this population.

Internationally, government policies need to address appropriate funding for early diagnosis, interventions, education and training for children and adults on the spectrum, as well as their parents, carers, communities and professionals actively involved in ASD provision across the lifespan.

Finally, and most importantly, the voices of children and adults with ASD need to inform development, provision and practice of quality programmes going forward.

References

American Psychiatric Association (1994) *Diagnostic and Statistical Manual of Mental Disorders, DSM-IV*. Washington, DC: American Psychiatric Association.

American Psychiatric Association (APA) (2013) *Diagnostic and Statistical Manual of Mental Disorders, Fifth Edition*. Washington, DC: American Psychiatric Association.

Asperger, H. (1944) Problems of infantile ASD. *Communication, 13*, 45–52.

Avila, L., Chiviacowsky, S., Wulf, G. and Lewthwaite, R. (2012) Positive-comparative feedback enhances motor learning in children. *Psychology of Sport and Exercise, 13*, 849–853.

Bachman, J.E. and Sluyter, D. (1988) Reducing inappropriate behaviours of developmentally disabled adults using antecedent aerobic dance exercises. *Research in Developmental Disabilities, 9*, 73–83.

Baird, G., Simonoff, E., Pickles, A., Chandler, S., Loucas, T., Meldrum, D. and Charman, T. (2006) Prevalence of disorders of the autism spectrum in a population cohort of children in South Thames: the Special Needs and Autism Project (SNAP). *The Lancet, 368*(9531), 210–215.

Bandini, L.G., Gleason, J., Curtin, C., Lividini, K., Anderson, S.E., Cermak, S.A. and Must, A. (2013) Comparison of physical activity between children with autism spectrum disorders and typically developing children. *Autism, 17*(1), 44–54.

Bandura, A. (1986) *Social Foundations of Thought and Action: A Social Cognitive Theory*. Englewood Cliffs, NJ: Prentice-Hall.

Bardid, F., Lenoir, M., Huyben, F., De Martelaer, C., Jan Seghers, J., Goodway, D. and Deconinck, F. (2017) The effectiveness of a community-based fundamental motor skill intervention in children aged 3–8 years: Results of the 'Multimove for Kids' project. *Journal of Science and Medicine in Sport, 20*(2), 184–189.

Barnett, L., Beurden, V., Morgan, P., Brooks, L.O. and Beard, J. (2009) Childhood motor skill proficiency as a predictor of adolescent physical activity. *Journal of Adolescent Health, 44*, 252–259.

131

Bellows, L., Davies, P., Courtney, J., Gavin, J., Johnson, S. and Boles, R. (2017) Motor skill development in low-income, at-risk preschoolers: A community-based longitudinal intervention study. *Journal of Science and Medicine in Sport, 20*(11), 997–1002.

Berkeley, S.L., Zittel, L.L., Pitney, L.V. and Nichols, S.E. (2001) Locomotor and object control skills of children diagnosed with ASD. *Adapted Physical Activity Quarterly, 18*(4), 405–416.

Bernstein, N. (1967) *The Co-Ordination and Regulation of Movement.* Oxford: Pergamon Press.

Block, M.E. (2000) *A Teacher's Guide to including Children with Disabilities in General Physical Education* (2nd edn). Baltimore, MD: Paul H. Brookes.

Bloom, B.S., Engelhart, M.D., Furst, E.J., Hill, W.H. and Krathwohl, D.R. (1956) *Taxonomy of Educational Objectives: The Classification of Educational Goals. Handbook I: Cognitive Domain.* New York: David McKay Company.

Bond, C., Colea, M., Crook, H., Fletcher, J., Lucanz, J. and Noblea, J. (2007) The development of the Manchester Motor Skills Assessment (MMSA): An initial evaluation. *Educational Psychology in Practice, 23*(4), 363–379.

Bondy, A. and Frost, L. (1994) The Picture Exchange Communication System. *Focus on Autistic Behaviour, 9,* 1–19.

Bondy, A. and Frost, L. (2001) The Picture Exchange Communication System. *Behaviour Modification, 25,* 725–744.

Bremer, E. and Lloyd, M. (2016) School-based fundamental-motor-skill intervention for children with autism-like characteristics: An exploratory study. *Adapted Physical Activity Quarterly, 33*(1), 66–88.

Bremer, E., Balogh, R. and Lloyd, M. (2014) Effectiveness of a fundamental motor skill intervention for 4-year-old children with autism spectrum disorder: A pilot study. *Autism, 19*(8), 980–991.

Bruininks, R.H. (1978) *The Bruininks–Osteretsky Test of Motor Proficiency.* Circle Pines, MN: American Guidance Service.

Bruininks, R.H. and Bruininks, B.D. (2005) *Test of Motor Proficiency* (2nd edn). Circle Pines, MN: AGS Publishing.

Carlson, S.A., Fulton, J.E., Schoenborn, C.A. and Loustalot, F. (2010) Trend and prevalence estimates based on the 2008 Physical Activity Guidelines for Americans. *American Journal of Preventive Medicine, 39*(4), 305–313.

Cattuzzo, M., Henrique, R., Hervaldo, A., Ré, N., de Oliveira, I.S., Machado Melo, B., De Sousa Moura, M., Cappato de Araújo, R. and Stodden, D. (2016) Motor competence and health related physical fitness in youth: A systematic review. *Journal of Science and Medicine in Sport, 19*(2), 123–129.

Celeberti, D.A., Bobo, H.E., Kelly, K.S., Harris, S.L. and Handleman, J.S. (1997) The differential and temporal effects of antecedent exercise on the self-stimulatory behaviour of a child with autism. *Research in Developmental Disabilities, 18,* 139–150.

Centers for Disease Control and Prevention (CDC) (2009) Prevalence of autism spectrum disorder among children aged 8 years. Autism and Developmental Disabilities Monitoring Network, 11 sites, United States, 2006. *MMWR, 58*, SS.10.

Chambers, M. and Sugden, D. (2006) *Early Years Movement Skills: Description, Diagnosis and Intervention*. Hoboken, NJ: Wiley.

Constantino, J. and Gruber, D. (2005) *Social Responsiveness Scale*. Los Angeles, CA: Western Psychological Services.

Crawford, S. and Dorney, S. (2011) Examining the effects of a parent led physical activity intervention on the fundamental movement skills of children with ASD. Poster presented at AIESEP, University of Limerick, Ireland.

Crawford, S., MacDonncha, C. and Smyth, P.J. (2007) An examination of current provision and practice of adapted physical activity for children with disabilities and the subsequent application of an adapted physical activity intervention programme for children with ASD and co-occurring learning disabilities. PhD thesis, University of Limerick, Ireland.

Crawford, S., O'Reilly, R. and Flanagan, N. (2012) Examining current provision, practice and experience of initial teacher training providers in Ireland preparing pre service teachers for the inclusion of students with special education needs in physical education classes. *European Journal of Adapted Physical Activity, 5*(2), 7–16.

Crawford, S., MacDonncha, C. and Smyth, P.J. (2013) Examining fundamental movement skills and social responsiveness of children with autism following a randomized physical activity intervention. *US-China Education Review B, 3*(8), 593–602.

Crawford, S., Lee, M. and Fitzpatrick, T. (2015) Exploring the use of mobile digital technology and iPod Touches in physical education. In: *International Handbook of Digital Technology in Teaching and Learning in Higher Education*. India: Springer.

Department of Education and Science (2001) *Educational Provision and Support for Persons with Autistic Spectrum Disorders: The Report of the Task Force on Autism*. Retrieved 16 April 2018 from www.sess.ie/sites/default/files/Autism%20Task%20Force%20Report.pdf

Dillenburger, K., Keenan, M., Gallagher, S. and McElhinney, M. (2004) Parent education and home-based behaviour analytic intervention: An examination of parent's perceptions of outcome. *Journal of Intellectual and Developmental Disabilities, 29*, 119–130.

Dunlap, G. (1984) The influence of task variation and maintenance tasks on the learning and affect of autistic children. *Journal of Experimental Child Psychology, 37*, 41–64.

Elsabbagh, M., Divan, G., Koh, Y.-J., Kim, Y.S., Kauchali, S., Marcín, C., Montiel-Nava, C., Patel, V., Paula, C.S., Wang, C., Yasamy, M.T. and Fombonne, E. (2012) Global prevalence of autism and other pervasive developmental disorders. *Autism Research, 5*, 160–179.

Erba, H.W. (2000) Early intervention programmes for children with ASD: Conceptual frameworks for implementation. *American Journal of Orthopsychiatry, 70*, 82–94.

Ericsson, I. (2011) Effects of increased physical activity on motor skills and marks in physical education: An intervention study in school years 1 through 9 in Sweden. *Physical Education Sport Pedagogy, 16*, 313–329.

Ericsson, K., Krampe, R. and Tesch-Römer, C. (1993) The role of deliberate practice in the acquisition of expert performance. *Psychological Review, 100*(3): 363–406.

Flanagan, H., Perry, A. and Freeman, N. (2012) Effectiveness of large scale community based intensive intervention: A waitlist comparison study comparing outcomes and predictors. *Research in Autism Spectrum Disorders, 6*, 673–682.

Fitts P. and Posner, M. (1967) *Human Performance.* Belmont, CA: Brooks/Cole Pub. Co.

Folio, M.R. and Fewell, R.R. (1983) *Peabody Developmental Motor Scales and Activity Cards.* Allen, TX: DLM Teaching Resources.

Folio, M.R. and Fewell, R.R. (2000) *Peabody Developmental Motor Scales – 2.* Austin, TX: Pro-Ed Inc.

Folstein, S. and Rutter, M. (1977) Infantile ASD: A genetic study of 21 twin pairs. *Journal of Child Psychology and Psychiatry, 18*, 297–231.

Frith, U. (2003) *ASD: Explaining the Enigma* (2nd edn). Oxford: Blackwell Press.

Gallahue, D.L. and Donnelly, F.C. (2003) *Developmental Physical Education for All Children* (4th edn). Champaign, IL: Human Kinetics.

Gallahue, D. and Ozmun, J. (2002) *Understanding Motor Development* (5th edn). Dubuque, IA : McGraw-Hill.

Gallahue, D. and Ozmun, J. (2006) *Understanding Motor Development* (6th edn). Boston, MA: McGraw Hill.

Gentile, A.M. (1972) A working model of skill acquisition with application to teaching. *Quest, 17*, 3–23.

Gentile, A.M. (2000) Skill acquisition: Action, movement, and neuromotor processes. In: J.H. Carr and R.D. Shepherd (eds), *Movement Science Foundations for Physical Therapy* (2nd edn). (pp. 111–187). Rockville, MD: Aspen.

Ghaziuddin, M. and Butler, E. (1998) Clumsiness in ASD and Asperger's syndrome: A further report. *Journal of Intellectual Disability Research, 42*, 43–48.

Grandin, T. (1996) *Thinking in Pictures and Other Reports from my Life with ASD.* New York: Vintage Books.

Heflin, L. and Alberto, P.A. (2001) ABA and instructions of students with ASD spectrum disorders: Introduction to the special series. *Journal of ASD and Developmental Disorders, 25*, 459–480.

Henderson S.E. and Sugden, D.A. (1992) *Movement Assessment Battery for Children.* London: Psychological Corporation.

Henderson, S. and Sugden, D. (2007) *Ecological Intervention for Children with Movement Difficulties.* London: Harcourt Assessment.

Henderson, S.E., Sugden, D.A. and Barnett, A.L. (2007a) *Movement Assessment Battery for Children – 2.* London: Pearson Education.

Henderson, S.E., Sugden, D.A. and Barnett, A.L. (2007b) *Movement Assessment Battery for Children – 2. Examiner's Manual.* London: Harcourt Assessment.

Henrique, R.S., Ré, A.H.N., Stodden, D.F., Fransen, J. et al. (2016) Association between sports participation, motor competence and weight status: A longitudinal study. *Journal of Science and Medicine in Sport, 19*(10), 825–829.

Hilton, C., Wente, L., LaVesser, P., Ito, M., Reed, C. and Herzberg, G. (2007) Relationship between motor skill impairment and severity in children with Asperger's syndrome. *Research in Autism Spectrum Disorders, 1*, 339–349.

Howlin, P. (1997) *Autism: Preparing for Adulthood.* London: Routledge.

Jasmin, E., Couture, M., McKinley, P., Reid, G., Fombonne, E. and Gisel, E. (2009) Sensori-motor and Daily Living Skills of Preschool Children with Autism Spectrum Disorders. *Journal of Autism and Developmental Disorders, 39*(2), 231–241.

Jordan, R., Jones, G. and Murray, D. (1998) *Educational Interventions for Children with ASD: A Review of Recent and Current Research.* Sudbury: Department for Education and Employment.

Kalaja, S.P., Jaakkola, T.T., Liukkonen, J.O. and Digelidis, N. (2012) Development of junior high school students' fundamental movement skills and physical activity in a naturalistic physical education setting. *Physical Education and Sport Pedagogy, 17*(4), 411–428.

Kanner, L. (1943) Autistic disturbances of affective contact. *Nervous Child, 2*, 217–250. In L. Wing (ed.) (2002) *The Autistic Spectrum: A Guide for Parents and Professionals.* London: Robinson.

Kazdin, A.E. and Hartmann, D.P. (1978) The simultaneous treatment design. *Behaviour Therapy, 9*, 912–922.

Kern, L., Koegel, R. and Dunlap, G. (1984) The influence of vigorous versus mild exercise on autistic stereotyped behaviours. *Journal of ASD and Developmental Disorders, 14*, 57–67.

Ketcheson, L., Hauck, J. and Ulrich, D. (2016) The effects of an early motor skill intervention on motor skills, levels of physical activity, and socialization in young children with autism spectrum disorder: A pilot study. *Autism, 21*(4), 481–492.

Koegel, R.L. and Koegel, L.K. (2006) *Pivotal Response Treatments for ASD: Communication, Social, and Academic Development.* Baltimore, MD: Paul H. Brookes.

Koegel, R.L., Dyer, K. and Bell, L.K. (1987) The influence of child-preferred activities on autistic children's social behavior. *Journal of Applied Behavior Analysis 20,* 243–252.

Koegel, R.L., Koegel, L.K. and Carter, C.M. (1999) Pivotal teaching interactions for children with ASD. *School Psychology Review 28,* 576–594.

Kozub, F.M. (2001) Adapted physical activity programming within the family – the family systems theory. *Palaestra, 17*(3), 30–38.

Landa, R. (2008) ASD spectrum disorders in the first 3 years of life. In: B.K. Shapiro and P.J. Accardo (eds) *ASD Frontiers: Clinical Issues and Innovations* (pp.97–123). Baltimore, MD: Paul H. Brookes.

Lewthwaite, R. and Wulf, G. (2010) Social-comparative feedback affects motor skill learning. *Quarterly Journal of Experimental Psychology, 63*(4), 738–749.

Liu, T. and Breslin, C.M. (2013) Fine and gross motor performance of the MABC-2 by children with autism spectrum disorder and typically developing children. *Research in Autism Spectrum Disorders, 7,* 1244–1249.

Lloyd, M., MacDonald, M. and Lord, C. (2013) Motor skills of toddlers with autism spectrum disorders. *Autism: International Journal of Research and Practice, 17,* 133–146.

Logan, S.W., Webster, E.K., Lucas, W.A. and Robinson, L.E. (2011) Effectiveness of a student-led motor skill intervention in preschool children. *Research Quarterly for Exercise and Sport, 82*(Suppl.): A31, 1–11.

Lovaas, O.I. (1987) Behavioural treatment and normal educational and intellectual functioning in young autistic children. *Journal of Consulting and Clinical Psychology, 55,* 3–9.

Lovaas, O.I. (1993) The development of a treatment-research project for developmentally disabled and autistic children. *Journal of Applied Behavior Analysis, 26,* 617–630.

Lubans, D.R., Morgan, P.J., Cliff, D.P. et al. (2010) Fundamental movement skills in children and adolescents: Review of associated health benefits. *Sports Medicine, 40,* 1019–1035.

MacDonald, M., Esposito, P. and Ulrich, D. (2011) The physical activity patterns of children with ASD. *BMC Research Notes, 4*(1), 422.

MacDonald, M., Lord, C. and Ulrich, D.A. (2013) The relationship of motor skills and social communicative skills in school-aged children with autism spectrum disorder. *Adapted Physical Activity Quarterly, 30,* 271–282.

Magill, R.A. (1993) Augmented feedback in skill acquisition. In: R.N. Singer, M. Murphy and L.K. Tennant (eds) *Handbook of Research on Sport Psychology* (pp.193–212). New York: Macmillan.

Magill, R. (2011) *Motor Learning and Control Concepts and Applications* (9th edn). New York: McGraw-Hill.

Manjiviona, J. and Prior, M. (1995) Comparison of Asperger syndrome and high functioning autistic children on a test of motor impairment. *Journal of ASD and Developmental Disorders, 25,* 23–29.

Maurice, C. (1993) *Let Me Hear Your Voice: A Family's Triumph over ASD.* London: Robert Hale.

McGimsey, J.F. and Favell, J.E. (1988) The effects of increased physical exercise on disruptive behaviour in retarded persons. *Journal of Autism and Developmental Disorders, 18,* 167–179.

Mesibov, G.B. and Shea, V. (2003) *The Culture of ASD: From Theoretical Understanding to Educational Practice.* London: Fulton.

Mesibov, G.B., Browder, D.M. and Kirkland, C. (2002) Using individualized schedules as a component of positive behavioral support for students with developmental disabilities. *Journal of Positive Behavior Interventions, 4,* 73–79.

Morin, B. and Reid, G. (1985) A quantitative and qualitative assessment of autistic individuals on selected motor tasks. *Adapted Physical Activity Quarterly, 2*(1), 43–55.

Mouratidis A., Lens, W. and Vansteenkiste, M. (2010) How you provide corrective feedback makes a difference. *Journal of Sport & Exercise Psychology, 32,* 619–637.

Myles, B.S. (2001) Practical solutions for teaching children and youth with autism and Asperger syndrome. *MRDD Express, 12*(1), 1–6.

National Alliance for Autism Research (2005) About autism. Retrieved 13 February 2016 from www.naar.org/aboutaut/whatis.htm.

National Autistic Society (2000) *The ASD Handbook.* London: National Autistic Society.

Neely, L., Rispoli, M.,Camargo, S., Davis, H. and Boles M. (2013) The effect of instructional use of an iPad on challenging behaviour and academic engagement for two students with autism. *Research in Autism Spectrum Disorders, 7,* 509–516.

Neidert, P.L., Iwata, B.A. and Dozier, C.L. (2005) Treatment with multiply controlled problem behavior with procedural variations of differential reinforcement. *Exceptionality, 13*(1), 45–53.

Newman, B., Needelman, M., Reinecke, D.R. and Roebek, A. (2002) The effect of providing choices on skill acquisition and competing behaviour of children with ASD during discrete trial instruction. *Behavioural Interventions, 17,* 31–41.

NSW Department of Education and Training (2000) *Get skilled: Get active.* Sydney: Curriculum Support Directorate.

O'Connor, J., French, R. and Henderson, H. (2000) Use of physical activity to improve behaviour of children with autism: Two for one benefits. *Palaestra, 16*(3), 22–26, 28-29.

O'Keeffe, S., Harrison, A.J. and Smyth, P.J. (2007) Transfer or specificity? *Physical Education and Sport Pedagogy, 12,* 89–102.

Okely, A., Booth, M. and Patterson, J. (2001) Relationship of physical activity to fundamental movement skills among adolescents. *Medicine and Science in Sports and Exercise, 33*(11), 1899–1904.

Okely, A., Booth, M. and Cheyet, T. (2004) Relationships between body compositions and fundamental movement skills among children and adolescents. *Research Quarterly for Exercise and Sport, 75*(3), 238–247.

Pan, C.Y., Tsai, C.L. and Chu, C.H. (2009) Physical activity and self-determined motivation of adolescents with and without ASD spectrum disorders in inclusive physical education. *Research in ASD Spectrum Disorders, 5*, 733–741.

Payne, V.G. and Isaacs, L.D. (2002) *Human Motor Development: A Lifespan Approach* (5th edn). Boston, MA: McGraw-Hill.

Payne, V.G. and Isaacs, L.D. (2011) *Human Motor Development: A Lifespan Approach* (8th edn). Boston, MA: McGraw-Hill.

Powers, S., Thibadeau, S. and Rose, K. (1992) Antecedent exercise and its effects on self-stimulation. *Behavioural Residential Treatment, 7*, 15–22.

Prupas, A. and Reid, G. (2001) Effects of exercise frequency on stereotypic behaviors of children with developmental disabilities. *Education and Training in Mental Retardation and Developmental Disabilities, 36*, 196–206.

Quill, K.A. (2000) *Do-Watch-Listen-Say: Social Communication Intervention for Children with Autism.* Baltimore, MA: Paul H. Brookes.

Reid, G. and Collier, D. (2002) Motor behaviour and the autistic spectrum disorders – introduction. *Palaestra, 18*(4), 20–27, 44.

Reid, G. and O'Connor, J. (2003) The ASD spectrum disorders: Activity selection, assessment and program organization. *Palaestra, 19*(1), 20–27, 58.

Reid, G., O'Connor, J. and Lloyd, M. (2003) The autistic spectrum disorders: Physical activity instruction – part III. *Palaestra, 19*(2), 20–26, 47–48.

Riggen, K.J., Ulrich, D.A. and Ozmun, J.C. (1990) Reliability and concurrent validity of the Test of Motor Impairment – Henderson Revision. *Adapted Physical Activity Quarterly, 7*(3): 249–258.

Ring, E. (2006) Review of evaluation of ASD provision in Irish schools. Dublin: Department of Education and Science.

Rose, D.J. and Heath, E.M. (1990) Development of a diagnostic instrument for evaluating tennis serving performance. *Perceptual and Motor Skills, 71*, 355–363.

Sandt, D. and Frey, G. (2005) Comparison of physical activity levels between children with and without autistic spectrum disorders. *Adapted Physical Activity Quarterly, 22*, 146–159.

Schleien, S., Krotee, T., Kelterborn, B. and Schermer, D. (1987) The effect of integrating children with ASD into a physical activity and recreational setting. *Therapeutic Recreation Journal, 21*, 52–62.

Schopler, E. and Mesibov, G.B. (1986) *Social Behaviour in Autism.* New York: Plenum Press.

Schopler, E. and Mesibov, G.B. (2000) International priorities for developing ASD services via the TEACCH model – 1 – guest editor's introduction – cross-cultural priorities in developing ASD service. *International Journal of Mental Health, 29,* 3–21.

Schultheis, S., Boswell, B. and Decker, J. (2000) Successful physical activity programming for students with ASD. *Focus on ASD and other Developmental Disabilities, 15*(3), 159–162.

Seal, B.C. and Bonvillian, J.D. (1997) Sign language and motor functioning in students with autistic disorder. *Journal of ASD and Developmental Disorders, 27,* 437–466.

Simpson, R.L. and Zionts, P. (1999) *Autism: Information and Resources for Professionals and Parents.* Austin, TX: Pro-Ed.

Skinner, B.F. (1953) *Science and Human Behaviour.* New York: Macmillan.

Staples, K.L. and Reid, G. (2010) Fundamental movement skills and autism spectrum disorders. *Journal of Autism and Developmental Disorders, 40,* 209–217.

Staples, K.L., Reid, G., Pushkarenko, K. and Crawford, S. (2011) Physically active living for individuals with ASD. In: J.L. Matson and P. Sturmey (eds) *International Handbook of Autism and Pervasive Developmental Disorders* (pp. 397–412). New York, NY: Springer.

Starkes, J.L., Deakin, J.M., Allard, F., Hodges, N.J. and Hayes, A. (1996) Deliberate practice in sports: What is it anyway? In: K.A. Ericsson (ed.) *The Road to Excellence: The Acquisition of Expert Performance in the Arts and Sciences, Sports, and Games* (pp.81–106). Hillsdale, NJ: Lawrence Erlbaum Associates, Inc.

Stott, D.H., Moyes, F.A. and Henderson, S.E. (1984) *The Test of Motor Impairment.* San Antonio, TX: The Psychological Corporation.

Teitelbaum, P., Teitelbaum, O., Nye, J., Fryman, J. and Maurer, R.G. (1998) Movement analysis in infancy may be useful for early diagnosis of ASD. *Proceedings of the National Academy of Sciences: Psychology, 95,* 1982–1987.

Todd, T. and Reid, G. (2006) Increasing physical activity in individuals with ASD. *Focus on ASD and Other Developmental Difficulties, 21*(3), 167–176.

Tsangaridou, N. and O'Sullivan, M. (1994) Using pedagogical reflective strategies to enhance reflection among preservice physical education teachers. *Journal of Teaching in Physical Education 14,* 13–23.

Tyler, K., MacDonald, M. and Menear, K. (2014) Physical activity and physical fitness of school-aged children and youth with autism spectrum disorders. *Autism Research and Treatment,* 312163. doi: 10.1155/2014/312163.

Ulrich, D. (1985) *Test of Gross Motor Development.* Austin, TX: Pro-Ed Inc.

Ulrich, D.A. (2000) *Test of Gross Motor Development* (2nd edn). Austin, TX: Pro-Ed Inc.

Vivanti, G., Hudry, K., Trembath, D., Barbaro, J., Richdale, A. and Dissanayake, C. (2013) Towards the DSM-5 criteria for ASD: Clinical, cultural and research implications. *Australian Psychologist, 48*, 258–261.

Weber, R.C. and Thorpe, J. (1992) Teaching children with autism through task variation in physical education. *Exceptional Children, 59*, 77–86.

Wilczynski, S., Green, G., Ricciardi, J., Boyd, B., Hume, A., Ladd, M., Rue, H. (2009) *National Standards Report: The National Standards Project: Addressing the Need for Evidence-based Practice Guidelines for Autism Spectrum Disorders.* Randolph: The National Autism Center.

Wing, L. (2002) *The Autistic Spectrum: A Guide for Parents and Professionals.* London: Robinson.

Wing, L. (1996) Autism Spectrum Disorder. Editorial. *British Medical Journal, 312*, 327–328.

World Health Organization (1992) *The ICD-10 classification of mental and behavioural disorders: Clinical descriptions and diagnostic guidelines.* Geneva: World Health Organization.

Wright. H. and Sugden, D. (1999) *Physical Education for All: Developing Physical Education in the Curriculum for Pupils with Special Educational Needs.* London: David Fulton.

About the Author

Dr Susan Crawford is a lecturer in sports studies and physical education at the School of Education, University College Cork, Ireland. She originally qualified as a registered general nurse, midwife, holistic and sports massage therapist, and returned to complete a BSc in sport and exercise science as a mature student. Susan practised for many years in these combined areas before undertaking her PhD at the University of Limerick in the area of fundamental movement skill development and social responsiveness for children with ASD (2004–2007), having been the recipient of a scholarship from the Irish Research Council for Science, Engineering and Technology. Susan has also completed postgraduate studies (certificate, diploma and Master's thesis in teaching and learning in higher education in University College Cork, 2008–2011) to complement her understanding and knowledge of current best practice in the field. In 2014, Susan received the President's Award for innovation in research and teaching, particularly in relation to driving the agenda of university–school–community collaboration to address inclusive practice. She became a Fulbright Scholar in 2015 for her work developing the use of Mobile Digital Technology to address motor development and impairment for individuals on the autistic spectrum. This was in collaboration with Professor William Bosl at the University of San Francisco. Susan received a Digital Champion Award from the National Teaching and Learning Forum for further refining this work in 2016. In 2017, Susan became a Social Entrepreneur Ireland Mentee and, with the support of the Health Action Zone, HSE, in Cork, has set up the 'getautismactive' website through this initiative. This programme is currently being rolled out in schools and communities throughout Ireland.

Susan's research interests lie in the areas of fundamental movement skill development with specific emphasis on ASD. She is also keenly interested in the areas of reflective practice and driving the agenda of quality university–school–community collaborations across these combined areas. She has presented her work and published both nationally and internationally. Her previous books include *ASD and Physical Activity: What Every Parent Needs to Know* and *Adapted Physical Activity Interventions for Children and Adults on the Spectrum*, both sponsored by the Health Action Zone, HSE, Cork, Ireland. Susan has also designed the Get ASD Active and Get ASD Aware programmes, which are both to be found on the www.getautismactive.com website.

Susan's greatest experience comes from being the mother of Tomás, a young man diagnosed with ASD and learning disabilities, epilepsy and ASD-related catatonia. Tomás has inspired Susan to follow and grow her interest and work in the area of ASD. Together they have completed half-marathons, and thousands of 10km runs, trail blazers and hikes around the world.

Index

143